My Life with Multiple Sclerosis

"It Looks the Way I Make It Look!"

by
Carol Ann White

MHB Publishing, LLC.
Chicago, IL

PUBLISHED BY MHB PUBLISHING, LLC
P.O. Box 2502
Calumet City, IL 60409-9998

Printed in the United States of America

First Printing, 2021

Editing by: Joyce Dunmore

Cover Design: Carol Ann White

Cover Art: Hand, Bridge, Bubble, Light by geralt ™ (Gerd Altmann) via Pixabay

ISBN: 9798757354408

Table of Contents

Dedication

This book is dedicated to the MS fighters, our families, friends, co-workers and caregivers. WE GOT THIS!!!

Also, I have a few Thank You's to give:
- To my husband, Carl White. You have been with me since the journey began; you have been my rock, my strength, my courage and my peace of mind when it seemed like I was losing my mind. Your love is invaluable to me; Thank You for loving me!!!

- To Brushella (no last name; I only know that she was the chaplain at the now closed Mercy Hospital here in Chicago): Thank You for the clarity, advice and options you blessed me with as we sat in the holding room waiting for our mammograms. Your perspective was invaluable to me, and the reason I chose to author this book.

"Multiple Sclerosis is a journey I never planned or asked for, but I chose to –
- ➢ Love Life
- ➢ Hate the Disease
- ➢ And FIGHT!!!"

- Anonymous

Introduction

Allow me to introduce myself: my name is Carol Ann White. I am a retired Chicago police officer, an author, publisher and owner of MHB Publishing, LLC., and I am a Life Detox Strategist. I am also a wife, lover, daughter, sister, aunt, cousin, friend, confidant, court advocate/community activist, Christian and choir member. I also have Multiple Sclerosis. That's a pretty full plate if I do say so myself!

Why did I give you this laundry list about me? Because all of these things made up who I was prior to my MS diagnosis, and they are still make up who I am *with MS*. Life as you know it to be doesn't stop, but it does change. What is important to understand is that *you have control over that change!* I am still retired, I still write, publish and run my company; I'm still married;

I still have my family and friends; and I still enjoy my activities. It's just that now, I enjoy them with a new set of health rules. I always keep in mind that this is my life, and I don't have to give it over to my Multiple Sclerosis; I can make my life look the way I want it to look!

Believe me - there are days that I just want to pull the covers over my head and hide from the world because my symptoms have flared up and I just don't want to face the day; I have had my share of breakdowns and pity parties. Living with a chronic illness is hard, and it can drain you emotionally as well as physically. So, on the days I feel drained, I give myself permission to power down and rest until I'm feeling better, and I tell Carl, my husband, to fend for himself because "today is not the day." And my husband, God bless him, kisses me on the cheek, tucks me in, and goes out to buy dinner.

But the one thing I constantly tell myself when I feel like this is that I am not entitled to stay in "pity party" mode! It is so easy to get trapped in despair and depression; my mother used to say, "Worry, stress, and fear are like quicksand to the spirit. The more you thrash around in them, the deeper you sink. To save yourself, you have to stop fighting and be still. Instead of looking at the mire that surrounds you, look up towards Heaven. And as you focus on your stillness, you just might see a tree branch within reach you can use to pull yourself out."[1]

It is for these reasons I chose to write **MY LIFE WITH MULTIPLE SCLEROSIS: It Looks the Way I Make It Look;** I wanted to offer the MS fighters a tree branch by easing their confusion in two ways: one, I wanted to let the fighters know that they are not fighting alone, and someone understands. And two, I wanted to give the MS fighters a collective resource of information to ease the stress, worry, fear and confusion that comes with dealing with our disease. I sincerely hope this helps you build your arsenal.

Addendum: There may be some issues with Multiple Sclerosis that I have not covered in this book. This is only because at this point in my journey I have not encountered nor experienced these symptoms. But I have given resources

---

[1] From the Foreword of Sage Sayings to Season the Soul by Maude Helen Baker

with which you can gain information and clarity for what has not been covered. There's always room for a sequel....

<u>References and Resources</u>

1. *Sage Sayings to Season the Soul by Maude Helen Baker* ©2017

Essay 1: What Does MS Look Like?

__MULTIPLE SCLEROSIS__: an autoimmune disease that attacks the myelin sheath around the nerves within the central nervous system. The result is that your body cannot effectively conduct messages between your brain and your body. (summary of various definitions)

Plainly put, your body mistakes the myelin for something bad, like a virus, and tries to protect the body from the intruder. The damaged myelin, for whatever reason, does not regenerate, so scars – lesions – form over the damage (sclerosis).[1] Since scar tissue does not conduct the nerve impulses, the result is there are gaps in the transmission of signals between

---

[1] Let's Talk About Multiple Sclerosis (MS) Causes by Patrick Sullivan, Medically Reviewed by Guillaume Lamotte, M.D. June 4, 2020.

the brain and the body; a short circuit, if you will.

The causes of MS are, at this time, still unknown, but here is what is known:

1. MS can occur at any age, but it is usually diagnosed between the ages of 20 and 40.
2. Women are 2 to 3 times more likely to suffer from MS, and 4 times more likely to get the most common form of MS (relapsing-remitting MS {RRMS}).
3. MS does not racially discriminate! Caucasians and African Americans are most at risk for getting MS, but all races are susceptible to MS.
4. Family History – if a parent or sibling has MS, you are more likely to get MS. MS, however, is not hereditary.
5. Environment, geography, low vitamin D levels, smoking, obesity, and infections all play a part in whether or not you can get MS.[2]

There are four types of Multiple Sclerosis:

---

[2] Let's Talk About Multiple Sclerosis (MS) Causes by Patrick Sullivan, Medically Reviewed by Guillaume Lamotte, M.D. June 4, 2020.

- **Clinically Isolated Syndrome (CIS).** The causes of this type of MS are due to inflammation or loss of the **myelin** within the body {**myelin** is a lipid-rich (fatty) substance that surrounds nerve cell axons (the nervous system's "wires") to insulate them and increase the rate at which electrical impulses, called action potentials, are passed along the axon[3]} but doesn't fulfill the criteria for Multiple Sclerosis. Clinically Isolated Syndrome can lead to other types of MS; however, nine times out of 10 people with CIS never develop beyond that.[4]

- **Relapsing Remitting MS (RRMS).** RRMS accounts for 88, 80 to 85% of initial diagnoses of multiple sclerosis. You have episodes of inflammatory activity and well-defined attacks of new or recurrent neurologic symptoms. Between symptoms,

---

[3] Myelin From Wikipedia, the free encyclopedia Pg. 1

[4] What do we know about the different types of MS? Medically reviewed by Deborah Weatherspoon, Ph.D., R.N., CRNA — Written by Jenna Fletcher on January 18, 2019 Pg. 2

a person with RRMS will experience full or partial recovery in between their episodes.[5]

- **Primary Progressive Multiple Sclerosis (PPMS).** This type is less common and accounts for only 10 to 15% of all these cases. The neurological function is impaired, and symptomology gets worse as the disease progresses.[6]

- **Secondary Progressive MS**. This is normally seen as the next stage of the disease for people who have the relapsing remitting multiple sclerosis. The 50% of the people with the RRMS will develop this secondary progressive within 10 years. And about 90% will do it after about 25 years. the difference between the secondary progressive and relapsing remitting is that Secondary progressive may or may not involve occasional relapses, minor

---

[5] What do we know about the different types of MS? Medically reviewed by Deborah Weatherspoon, Ph.D., R.N., CRNA — Written by Jenna Fletcher on January 18, 2019 Pg. 2
[6] Ibid., Pgs. 2 & 3

remissions, or plateaus, meaning the symptomology will continue to progress.[7] [8] Now that we have defined what it is, what it does, and what causes MS, let us talk about how it looks and feels:

1. Unexplained muscle stiffness and spams.
2. Muscle weakness and/or paralysis.
3. Tingling and numbness in the arms, legs, and face.
4. Fatigue.
5. Blurred and/or double vision.
6. Lack of coordination.
7. Trouble balancing.
8. Memory loss.
9. Urinary urgency/urinary incontinence/bowel incontinence.
10. Difficulty concentrating.
11. Depression.[9] [10]

---

[7] Multiple sclerosis From Wikipedia, the free encyclopedia Pg. 9

[8] What do we know about the different types of MS? Medically reviewed by Deborah Weatherspoon, Ph.D., R.N., CRNA — Written by Jenna Fletcher on January 18, 2019 Pgs. 2 & 3

[9] Multiple Sclerosis – Causes, Symptoms, and Treatment ©2021 (Editors' Choice), Pgs. 2 & 3

[10] What You Need to Know About Multiple Sclerosis by HealthyWomen Editors, 12 Nov 2020, Pg. 3

So... what is the look of Multiple Sclerosis? It is an autoimmune disease that, while they are doing a lot of research on MS, there are not a whole lot of answers. It can affect everyone, and anything can trigger it. MS looks like stiff muscles, frequent falls, and a complete change in your life. But there is a reality to face: your MS will look like - WHAT YOU MAKE IT LOOK LIKE!!! MS is not a death sentence unless you make it a death sentence! Between medicinal therapy, physical therapy, exercise, and dietary reconfiguration, you can have an excellent quality of life! I almost forgot about the most important therapy of all: connecting with other MS fighters (I refuse to use the words victim(s) of sufferer[s]) so you know you are not alone and there are people who understand your struggle. Here are a few that I personally found helpful:

- Above MS Website (www.abovems.com)
- The National Multiple Sclerosis Society (https://www.nationalmssociety.org)
- MultipleSclerosis.net Website (www.multiplesclerosis.net)

- My MS Team Website (https://www.mymsteam.com)
- Everyday Health Website (www.everydayhealth.com)
- More to MS Website (https://www.moretoms.com)

In the coming essays, I will be talking about all of these therapies with you. The more information you have about Multiple Sclerosis, the better equipped you are to fight!

References and Resources

1. *Let us Talk About Multiple Sclerosis (MS) Causes by Patrick Sullivan, June 4, 2020.* www.healthcentral.com

2. *Myelin from Wikipedia, the free encyclopedia Pg. 1* https://en.wikipedia.org/wiki/Myelin

3. *Multiple sclerosis From Wikipedia, the free encyclopedia* https://en.wikipedia.org/wiki/Multiple_sclerosis

4. *What do we know about the different types of MS? Medically reviewed by Deborah Weatherspoon, Ph.D., R.N., CRNA — Written by Jenna Fletcher on January 18, 2019* https://www.medicalnewstoday.com/articles/315320#treatment

5. *Multiple Sclerosis – Causes, Symptoms, and Treatment ©2021 (Editors' Choice)* https://wellnessbible.net/multiple-sclerosos-causes-symptoms-and-treatment/

6. *What You Need to Know About Multiple Sclerosis by HealthyWomen Editors of the HealthyWomen website, 12 Nov 2020* https://healthywomen.org/created-with-support/what-you-need-to-know-about-multiple-sclerosis

7. *Types of Multiple Sclerosis by Robin Madell, Medically Reviewed by Deborah Weatherspoon, Ph.D., R.N., CRNA Updated on April 8, 2019* https://www.healthline.com/health/multiple-sclerosis/types-of-ms#primaryprogressive

8. *16 Early Symptoms of Multiple Sclerosis by the Healthline Editorial Team, Medically Reviewed by Deborah Weatherspoon, Ph.D.,*

My Life with Multiple Sclerosis

R.N., CRNA, Updated on October 23, 2019 https://www.healthline.com/health/multiple-sclerosis/early-signs#other-symptoms

Essay 2: Sometimes My MS Wins

There are days when I can look my MS in the face and tell it, "Not today. We're good. We're going to be fine. We're going to make it through." And then there are days that my MS tells me, "I have control." And one of the ways my MS takes control is with spasms.

These spasms come across and there are days when I have little or no use of my right hand (being dominant right hand, this is very problematic). My muscles will not do what they are supposed to do because the nerve signals go haywire. The spasms come so frequently and sometimes are so intense that it just makes sitting an uncomfortable event for me. I also have nerve glitches; the best way to describe it is to say that it feels like someone is taking a live wire and putting to my skin every 10 to 15 seconds. It reminds me of when I was working for the Chicago Police Department; we had to go through taser certification training and had to be tased, so we knew what it felt like. There is no other way to describe it.

On the days my MS wins, it takes all effort for me to get anything accomplished. I don't look the way I would normally want to look. Because of the spasticity in my hand, I can't hold a makeup brush, I can't manipulate the mascara brush, and I can't hold my blush brush. I know I can work with my left hand, but my makeup looks crazy when I do. So, I don't put on makeup and go bare faced into the world. This is what MS can look like.

It is not pleasant, it is not pretty, but it is a reality that those of us with MS deal with every day! We have great days, but our MS lets us know what our limitations are, at least until we can get it under control.

My entire right side has been affected with my MS. I have a walker at this point to assist me with my walking. But on the days my MS wins, even with my walker, it feels like I'm walking through waist high water, and I cannot lift my right leg. It is physically draining. There's no other way to describe it.

For those that want to know more about Multiple Sclerosis and what it is like on a difficult day, I'm going to give you a couple of articles for your information. These articles are written by MS fighters for MS fighters, as well as for family and friends of MS fighters, and the caregivers for MS fighters. And even though you cannot physically help the MS fighter get through their challenging days, your ability to understand what their situation is will help more than you realize.

<u>References and Resources:</u>

Of Sandcastles and Breakdowns by Devin Garlit · December 21, 2020
<u>https://multiplesclerosis.net/living-with-ms/breakdowns-resilience/?fbclid=IwAR2k1WcRcBwT5j4hNpkziSz8EIH_PO3BiVNHeSCk5FpZ0a5S-ovmyJaALKg</u>

The Monsters Within Us by Calie Wyatt · February 16, 2021
<u>https://multiplesclerosis.net/living-with-ms/monster-parenting-frustration/?fbclid=IwAR2rHnXHSGADNJvhPA7DYUJHTCd9cGu0XjtXkRUS-eIJRao3-zSFHZsgCbo</u>

Identifying New MS Symptoms Feels Like Opening Pandora's Box by Calie Wyatt · February 9, 2021
<u>https://multiplesclerosis.net/living-with-ms/new-symptoms-fear-anxiety/?fbclid=IwAR1vPw2EEK8_ZBj4gydJOVjdplF3E29uoq_K8xLRWJH4eP4aF5vR0ogm0Yk</u>

Section 1: MS Symptoms

Chapter 3: Spasticity, Tingling, Numbness, & Pain

Every morning, for the past several months, I wake up to a spastic right leg! I have come to realize that the spasticity levels in my leg determine what kind of day I am going to have; a three to five second spasticity session usually means I will have an average day. BUT – if I have a violent, massive, Richter scale level episode lasting 10 to 15 seconds, it is a safe bet I am going to have a pretty lousy day….

It does not end there. I then have to get up and get myself ready for the day; this has become challenging because my knees become numb and tingly while I am preparing for my day (bathing, makeup, etc.), so I have to constantly sit down and wait for these sensations to pass. After a while, the numbness and tingling sensations turn into pain. I have to stop everything and allow my body to rest and relax. Suffice it to say, if I have to be somewhere at, say, 11:30 AM, I need to start getting ready around 7:00 AM (6:30 AM if I plan to eat)!

For me and my MS, the spasticity, numbness, tingling, and pain go hand in hand; it is rare that I will experience one symptom without another. How these symptoms affect other fighters with MS are as unique as every MS fighter. Our common thread is that these are the result of damage to our spinal cords because of our disease. It is time to look at each of these symptoms for what they are and how we can best control them.

Spasticity

Spasticity is considered one of the most common symptoms of Multiple Sclerosis (MS), referring to an increase of muscle tone and the inability of your muscles to relax; another way to say this is "the feeling of stiffness and a wide range of involuntary muscle spasms."[1]. Spasticity can be mild (a tightening of muscles) to severe (painful, uncontrollable spasms) and usually affect the extremities, most often the legs but can affect your arms, back, and joints.[2] [3]

There are five kinds of spasms that occur with MS:

- **Extensor:** Your limb stiffens, and you cannot move the joint.
- **Flexor:** Your limb bends toward your body.
- **Clonus:** Muscles jerk and twitch involuntarily.
- **Stiffness:** Muscles are slow to relax (the mildest of spasms).
- **The MS Hug:** The tiny muscles between your ribs spasm.[4]

Spasticity has a number of triggers, the most common of them being environment (too hot or

---

[1] Spasticity, the National Multiple Sclerosis Society website, Pg. 1
[2] Ibid., Pg. 1
[3] Spasticity as a Symptom of Multiple Sclerosis by Julie Stachowiak, PhD June 04, 2021 Pg.1
[4] Ibid., Pg. 2

too cold weather), stress, quick or sudden movements, irritating clothing, a full bladder, or an increase in internal temperature (such as a fever or excessive exercise).[5]

The treatments for spasticity depend on the types of spasms you experience, how severe the spasms are, how much pain they cause, and how you respond to medication. Oral medications (muscle relaxants) prescribed for spasticity are:

- Baclofen
- Zanaflex
- Neurotonin
- Benzodiazepines (e.g., Valium)
- Dantrium
- Magnesium[6]

Should these prove ineffective, there are other medical options such as:

- **Intrathecal Baclofen** – an implanted pump that injects Baclofen into the space

---

[5] Spasticity as a Symptom of Multiple Sclerosis by Julie Stachowiak, PhD June 04, 2021 Pg. 4

[6] Ibid.

of the spinal column that contains cerebrospinal fluid[7].

- **Botulinum toxin injections (Botox)** — these are effective in reducing muscle tone and improving passive function (for adults).[8]

The non-medicinal therapies are physical and occupational therapy, as well as avoiding your triggers as much as possible. Other therapies include yoga, massage, active movement and other methods.[9] [10]

Numbness and Tingling

These conditions are two of the most common – and frequent - conditions of MS. The sensations can be separated into four categories:

1. **Paresthesia:** The feeling of pins and needles, or a crawling sensation.
2. **Dysesthesia:** A burning sensation along the nerve that may change how you feel pressure.

---

[7] Spasticity as a Symptom of Multiple Sclerosis by Julie Stachowiak, PhD June 04, 2021 Pg. 4

[8] Ibid., Pg.5

[9] Ibid., Pg. 6

[10] MS Spasticity – what you need to know Overcoming Multiple Sclerosis Website Pg. 3

3. **Hyperpathia:** An increased sensitivity to pain.
4. **Anesthesia**: A complete loss of any sensation.[11]

Most cases of numbness and tingling will come and go, and the episodes for most only last for a short time. It should be noted, however, that there are no medications to specifically treat numbness and tingling.[12] Managing the pain associated with numbness and tingling can be done by movement, warm compresses, vitamin D (as an anti-inflammatory), massage, stretching/flexion exercises, and acupuncture. If the pain is severe, your doctor may prescribe anticonvulsants, antidepressants, or a combination of the two.[13]

It has been reported that about eighty percent (80%) of all MS warriors experience pain at some point in their MS journey[14]. Being able to identify what the source of your pain is will

---

[11] Symptom Series: Numbness and tingling, from the Above MS website Pg. 1

[12] Numbness and Tingling in Multiple Sclerosis from the Verywellhealth website, Pg. 4

[13] Symptom Series: Numbness and tingling, from the Above MS website, Pgs. 2 & 3

[14] What Kind of Pain Does Multiple Sclerosis Cause? Reviewed By: Sheetal DeCaria, M.D. Pg. 3

greatly help you develop a management plan for daily function and living.

References and Resources

1. *Spasticity, the National Multiple Sclerosis Society website*
https://www.nationalmssociety.org/Symptoms-Diagnosis/MS-Symptoms/Spasticity

2. *Spasticity as a Symptom of Multiple Sclerosis by Julie Stachowiak, PhD, Medically reviewed by Huma Sheikh, MD on June 04, 2021*
https://www.verywellhealth.com/spasticity-in-multiple-sclerosis-2440814

3. *MS Spasticity – what you need to know, from the Overcoming Multiple Sclerosis Website*
https://overcomingms.org/about-multiple-sclerosis/ms-symptoms/ms-spasticity

4. *Symptom Series: Numbness and tingling, from the Above MS website*
https://www.abovems.com/en_us/home/what-

is-ms/ms-symptoms/ms-numbness-tingling.html

5. *Numbness and Tingling in Multiple Sclerosis, from the Verywellhealth website* https://www.verywellhealth.com/numbness-tingling-in-ms-2440806

6. *What Kind of Pain Does Multiple Sclerosis Cause? Reviewed By: Sheetal DeCaria, M.D.* https://www.epainassist.com/nerves/what-kind-of-pain-does-multiple-sclerosis-cause

7. *Controlling spasticity by Lori De Milto, Momentum Magazine, Winter 2016–17* https://momentummagazineonline.com/controlling-spasticity/

8. *Numbness or Tingling, the National Multiple Sclerosis Society website* https://www.nationalmssociety.org/Symptoms-Diagnosis/MS-Symptoms/Numbness

9. *MS Numbness, Tingling & Pins and Needles, from the Overcoming Multiple Sclerosis Website* https://overcomingms.org/about-multiple-sclerosis/ms-symptoms/ms-numbness

Essay 4: Vertigo and Imbalance Issues

I remember, as a child, I loved going to the amusement parks and riding on the Tilt-A-Whirl and the Centripetal Force Rides (you know, that cylinder ride where you stood against the wall; it would spin, and the force built up by its speed would pin you to the wall?). I loved that feeling of being off-balance and dizzy! I look back now and realize I liked it because that feeling only came once, maybe twice a year and the feeling only lasted a short time, and I could enjoy the rest of my time at the amusement park.

Now, that I have Multiple Sclerosis and suffer with vertigo and imbalance issues, I have my own personal "tilt-a-whirl" going on in my head! The sensations are different as well. Along with the dizziness and imbalance, I sometimes feel like I am floating in space or water, followed by a crash landing to the floor. And, getting off this ride (or, at least getting it to slow down) takes a whole set of skills that I never thought I would have to acquire!!!

What Is Vertigo?

Vertigo, by definition, is "a condition in which you feel off-balance and dizzy, as if your surroundings are moving, spinning, or swaying."[1] You could experience these symptoms even if you are perfectly still. There are other symptoms connected with vertigo, such as feeling lightheaded or the sensation of passing out. You may also experience abnormal eye movements, loss of hearing, ringing in the ears, as well as an inability to concentrate.[2] This is caused by the lesions that develop on the brainstem or the spinal cord and disrupt the pathways of the signals that allow you to keep

---

[1] Vertigo (Dizziness, Spinning) MediResource Inc. 1996 – 2021 from the MedBroadcast Website, Pg. 1
[2] Vertigo from Bing search engine, data supplied by Focus Media

your balance.[3] [4] Another cause for vertigo is problems within the vestibular system in the ear.[5]

Vertigo can also be caused by other conditions, such as:

- Migraine
- Stroke
- Medication
- Bacteria
- Viruses Dehydration
- Stress
- Anxiety
- Blood Vessel Disease
- Problems with the inner ear
- Low blood pressure[6] [7]

How is Vertigo Treated?

---

[3] Dizziness and Vertigo in Multiple Sclerosis by Paul Frysh, Medically Reviewed by Neha Pathak, MD on August 10, 2020 on the WebMD Website, Pg. 2

[4] MS & vertigo: what you need to know from the Overcoming Multiple Sclerosis Website, Pg. 1

[5] Vertigo (Dizziness, Spinning) MediResource Inc. 1996 – 2021 from the MedBroadcast Website, Pg. 2

[6] Ibid., Pgs. 1 & 2

[7] Dizziness and Vertigo in Multiple Sclerosis by Paul Frysh, Medically Reviewed by Neha Pathak, MD on August 10, 2020 on the WebMD Website, Pg. 2

It is possible for vertigo to go away on its own. If it does not, the treatment of your vertigo is going to depend on what is causing your symptoms. Here are seven possible courses of treatment:

1. **Physical Therapy** – *Vestibular rehabilitation* uses eye and head movements, balance training, and other maneuvers to help your brain learn new ways to use your other senses to compensate for the vertigo.
2. **Canalith Repositioning (the Epley Maneuver)** – This method uses a series of special head and neck movements to move the crystals from the fluid-filled semicircular canals of your inner ear to a different area, so they can be absorbed into the body.
3. **Medication** – Depending upon the root cause of your vertigo and its length of duration (a few hours to a few days), your doctor will prescribe medication (the list is long....).
4. **Surgery** – This is NOT a common procedure; it may be required if a tumor or

injury is causing your symptoms. Other surgical procedures include:

- Canal Plugging – A bone plug is placed in an area of the inner ear to prevent the semicircular canals from responding to movements.
- Labyrinthectomy – the vestibular labyrinth in the bad ear is disabled, allowing the other ear to control balance.
- Shunt Surgery
- Plugging the leak in the inner ear.

5. **Injections** – Used in cases where patients have not responded to other treatments.

6. **Psychotherapy** – Helps patients identify negative behaviors and replace them with positive solutions.

7. **Treatment for an Underlying Problem** – People with MS, diabetes, Parkinson's disease, heart disease, diabetes and anemia may develop vertigo and need specific treatments to target these diseases.[8]

---

[8] Vertigo Treatment: Getting Rid of the Spins by Julie Marks, Medically Reviewed by Sanjai Sinha, MD Reviewed: March 1, 2018

What Does a Vertigo Episode Look/Feel Like?

Let me describe my first vertigo episode to you: It was August 2012, and I was working as a Chicago police officer on a one-man car. I received a call of a domestic disturbance with a possible firearm on scene. I arrive at the address and, as I start to walk to the front door, the sidewalk starts moving in a snake-like motion. I look at the woman in the doorway and she is moving in the same snake motion. I was terrified! What if the offender is combative? What if I have to take a shot and cannot focus enough to hit the right target? I am also thinking about the liability I have just become to my backup.... Thankfully, the offender fled the scene before my arrival, but I can barely focus on the caller's story because it hurts too much to hold my head up and I cannot make her face stop moving! After giving the caller information for any future incidents, I managed to get back to my car and sit down; the movements finally cease, and I get back to my duties.

At the end of my shift, while driving back to the station, the road begins moving in the snakelike motion. I fight with everything I have to make it, and thankfully I did. A couple of my fellow officers noticed my erratic walking and (after making sure I was sick and not inebriated) requested permission to take me home. That night I woke up to my bedroom spinning with no way for me to stop it. The next day my fiancé drove me to my doctor who immediately sent me to the emergency room for vertigo.

This is what vertigo feels like; thankfully, I have had great doctors and physical therapists that have helped me through my episodes. Vertigo is manageable, and life is still what you choose to make it.

References and Resources

1. *Vertigo (Dizziness, Spinning) MediResource Inc. 1996 – 2021 from the MedBroadcast Website* https://medbroadcast.com/condition/getconditi on/vertigo#

2. *Vertigo from Bing search engine, data supplied by Focus Media*

3. *Dizziness and Vertigo in Multiple Sclerosis by Paul Frysh, Medically Reviewed by Neha Pathak, MD on August 10, 2020 on the WebMD Website* https://www.webmd.com/multiple-sclerosis/multiple-sclerosis-dizziness-vertigo

4. *MS & vertigo: what you need to know from the Overcoming Multiple Sclerosis Website* https://overcomingms.org/about-multiple-sclerosis/ms-symptoms/ms-vertigo

5. *Vertigo Treatment: Getting Rid of the Spins by Julie Marks, Medically Reviewed by Sanjai Sinha, MD Reviewed: March 1, 2018* https://www.everydayhealth.com/signs-symptoms/vertigo/vertigo-treatment-getting-rid-spins/

6. *Canalith repositioning procedure By Mayo Clinic Staff* https://www.mayoclinic.org/tests-procedures/canalith-repositioning-procedure/about/pac-20393315

7. *Canal Partitioning Mercy Medical Center Website (Cedar Rapids, IA)* https://www.mercycare.org/services/ear-nose-and-throat/ear-care/ear-disorders/benign-paroxysmal-positional-vertigo-bppv/canal-partitioning/

Essay 5: MS Fatigue - Do Not Tell Me to "Take A Nap!!!"

I find more often these days that I am feeling the effects of one symptom of my MS: THE FATIGUE!!! I find that activities I used to in a brief period of time are taking twice or even three times the amount of time to accomplish. To be specific – preparing meals, cleaning my home, getting dressed; even taking my morning bath takes an enormous amount of time!!! Let me describe this to you: firstly, I must use a shower chair because I cannot stand for the time it takes to shower without my legs going into spasms. Then, after the shower, I must carefully get out of the tub and situate the chair close to the bathroom sink so that I can sit down when my legs go numb while I am standing brushing my teeth, doing my facial routine, and applying my makeup. What used to take a maximum of 20 minutes now takes 45 to 50 minutes – on a GOOD DAY. A meal that used to be prepared in 45 to 50 minutes may now take 2 to 3 hours. My daily activities now require a lot of planning and adjusting….

To understand the MS Fatigue, I need to explain how MS affects the nervous system. My best example is to say that the nervous system is like a phone charger cord. The wires (nerves) are encased in a protective sheath (myelin) which affords proper conduction to the device (the body). When you have MS, your immune system eats away at your cord's protective layer leaving holes; white blood cells form into scar tissue – sclera - over the hole (much like when you try to tape over damage to the charging cord). The problem with the tape is the same problem with the sclera – neither substance is meant for the conduction of the power going through either cord; you experience short circuits within this closed system. While you can throw away your charging cord because it is no longer in working condition, MS fighters must work with what they have, which is faulty conduction from our nerves to our muscles. Our bodies (and our brains) must work much harder to do everything!!!

There are some people in your circle that are not going to understand the differences between MS fatigue and regular fatigue and will not understand why you just can't "take a nap" to recharge. I wouldn't be too hard on them because we MS fighters may still be learning them as well. It is more than just being tired because MS Fatigue:

- Tends to worsen as the day progresses.
- Appears more easily and more suddenly than ordinary fatigue.
- Is more severe than 'ordinary' fatigue.
- Tends to be aggravated by heat and humidity.
- Is more likely to interfere with daily activities than 'ordinary' fatigue.[1]

Because of these differences between MS Fatigue and 'ordinary' fatigue, our recharge period is going to be a lot longer. Think of

---

[1] Fatigue: An Invisible Symptom of Multiple Sclerosis (MSIF: MS International Foundation), Pg. 2

yourself as a battery that has lost all its charge; everything stops. And your recharge time depends upon whether you chose to recharge when it was necessary or if you worked yourself to the point of exhaustion (physically or mentally) ....[2]

So, how can you avoid MS Fatigue? To be honest, at this point of my MS journey, I can only give you the advice I received from my physical therapist: DO A LITTLE, REST A LITTLE. That's right, you now must plan every event in your day! Not only that, you also must plan to minimize what you do in a day. For example, one day I had to go to the hospital for an MRI. This meant getting bathed, dressed, preparing breakfast, getting to the hospital, walking to and through the orthopedic center to get the MRI, then walking back to the car and going home (do not worry, my husband drove). My husband has accepted the fact that, after I have a day like this, I am not going to stand up and cook dinner!!! He can look at me and see that I am completely wiped out; I look defeated and tired,

---

[2] Making information on MS fatigue accessible to all, updated March 3, 2021 (MSIF: MS International Foundation), Pg. 2

my knees and ankles have a numbing sensation that is insane, and I just want and need to rest for as long as it takes for these feelings to go away. We have take-out on days like this!

I found the MS International Foundation website (www.msif.org) during my research and they have several items that can help you identify and handle MS Fatigue. The first is the "Fatigue: An Invisible Symptom of MS" guide.[3] They also have the Fatigue Diary[4] in a PDF as well as the Word version of the Fatigue Diary.[5] With these tools you can better understand, as well as document, your MS Fatigue.

Share this information with your close family and friends. They need to know what you, and they, are going to be dealing with. Every fighter can use a well-equipped army that will not tell you to 'take a nap, you will be okay'!

---

[3] The "Fatigue: An Invisible Symptom of MS" guide
[4] The Fatigue Diary template (PDF)
[5] The Fatigue Diary template (Word)

<u>Resources and References</u>

1. *Fatigue: An Invisible Symptom of Multiple Sclerosis from the MS International Federation website Last updated: 3rd March 2021* https://www.msif.org/about-ms/symptoms-of-ms/fatigue/

2. *Making information on MS fatigue accessible to all, updated March 3, 2021* (MSIF: MS International Foundation) https://www.msif.org/about-ms/symptoms-of-ms/fatigue/

3. *Fatigue: An Invisible Symptom of MS Booklet* http://www.msif.org/wp-content/uploads/2021/02/MS-FATIGUE-BOOKLET-DIGITAL.pdf

4. *The Fatigue Diary template (PDF)* http://www.msif.org/wp-content/uploads/2020/04/FATIGUE-DIARY-PRINT.pdf

5. *The Fatigue Diary template (Word)* http://www.msif.org/wp-content/uploads/2020/04/FATIGUE-DIARY.docx

6. *Managing and Preventing MS Fatigue by Colleen Doherty, MD, Medically Reviewed by Claudia Chaves, MD April 17, 2020* https://www.verywellhealth.com/fatigue-in-multiple-sclerosis-4042971

7. *Multiple Sclerosis: Fatigue* https://www.abovems.com/en_us/home/what-is-ms/ms-symptoms/fatigue.html

8. *MS Fatigue: What to Know Medically reviewed by Seunggu Han, M.D. — Written by Jacquelyn Cafasso on March 14, 2019* https://www.healthline.com/health/multiple-sclerosis/ms-fatigue

Essay 6: Foot Drop - What It Is, What It Does, and How to Cope

Imagine walking along and suddenly you discover (via a stumble and fall) you are not able to plant your foot normally; you do not have that heel-to-toe motion going on. You think it is a fluke, until you discover that this is not going away. Or, you begin to notice you have trouble curling or flexing your toes, as well as some numbness/weakness in them as well. Then you discover that you cannot flex or rotate your ankle as you once could. The combination of all this frightens you, so you speak to your neurologist who, after examining the way you walk and evaluates your muscle strength, gives you their diagnosis of Foot Drop (or drop foot).

And... so begins your journey of shoe inserts, AFO (ankle/foot orthotics) braces, canes, walkers, and countless hours of physical therapy. Your life is going to change from this point forward. In this chapter we will discuss what Foot Drop is, what causes it, how it is diagnosed, and the treatments available for Drop Foot.

The Definition of Foot Drop

Let us start at the beginning. What is **Foot Drop?** One particularly good definition is given in the article *Foot Drop (Feet Muscle Weakness) by Dr. Chris* on the Healthyhype.com website:

> Foot drop refers to difficulty in lifting the front part of the foot, due to weakness of the ankle and toe.... Foot drop occurs when the muscles, nerves or parts of the brain coordinating the movement of the foot is damaged or diseased. This may result in dragging the front of

the foot on the ground while walking.[1]

In order to compensate for the lack of heel-to-toe gait and clearing the floor while walking, you may find yourself walking one of two ways in order to compensate: you may lift your leg higher from the hip (steppage gait)[2] or swing your leg around your body (circumduction).[3]

The Causes of Foot Drop

The one thing you must understand about Foot Drop is that this IS NOT A DISEASE; it is a symptom of an underlying problem with a nerve, muscle, or anatomical structure. It is caused by a weakness or paralysis of the muscles involved with lifting the foot. There are three major reasons for this condition:

    1. Nerve Damage:

---

[1] Foot Drop (Feet Muscle Weakness) Posted by Dr. Chris Pg. 1
[2] Drop Foot: symptoms, causes and treatments Written by Dr. Bob Baravarian, DPM, FACFAS Foot and Ankle Surgeon and Director of University Foot and Ankle Institute updated 8/11/2021 Pg. 1
[3] Ibid. Pg.1

- Injury or compression to the peroneal nerve (located behind the outer part of your knee)
- Injury or damage to the sciatic nerve where it originates from the spine
- Certain diseases (i.e., diabetes)

2. Nerve or Muscle Disorders
   - Cerebral Palsy
   - Muscular Dystrophy
   - Polio
   - Charcot-Marie-Tooth Disease

3. Nervous System Disorders
   - Amyotrophic Lateral Sclerosis (ALS/Lou Gehrig's Disease)
   - Multiple Sclerosis
   - Strokes[4]

How Is Foot Drop Diagnosed?

The first way to diagnose Foot Drop is simple: your doctor and/or neurologist watches you walk. The abnormal gait of Foot Drop is easily detectable. You will also be evaluated for muscle weakness in the legs, numbness on top of your

---

[4] Drop Foot: symptoms, causes and treatments Written by Dr. Bob Baravarian, DPM, FACFAS Foot and Ankle Surgeon and Director of University Foot and Ankle Institute updated 8/11/2021 Pgs.1 & 2

foot, toes, and shin. In the event your neurologist thinks there is an underlying cause (such as nerve compression tumor or cyst), there will be more in-depth testing to identify the location of the problem:

1. X-rays
2. Ultrasounds (2D images)
3. CT scans
4. MRI's
5. Electromyography (EMG) (electrical activity in the muscles)
6. Nerve Conduction Velocity Studies (speed of neural impulses)[5] [6]

Treatments for Foot Drop

There are five (5) ways to treat Foot Drop:

1. **Devices** – this could consist of wearing a splint, using an AFO (ankle/foot/orthosis) to hold your foot in its proper position while walking, or wearing a brace on your ankle and foot. These devices usually are worn in

---

[5] Foot Drop (Feet Muscle Weakness) Posted by Dr. Chris, Pgs. 3 & 4

[6] Drop Foot: symptoms, causes and treatments Written by Dr. Bob Baravarian, DPM, FACFAS Foot and Ankle Surgeon and Director of University Foot and Ankle Institute updated 8/11/2021 Pg. 2

your shoe (some of these devices may require a shoe with more depth). They do have several other devices that fit on the outside of your shoe. The device I am currently using is the Xtern® by TurboMed Orthotics™.[7] I enjoy this far more than the AFO's I had to wear in my shoes, and it allows for greater movement in my ankle and a far more natural walking gait. They have other alternative devices that allow you the freedom of being able to wear different shoe styles.

2. **Physical Therapy** – this is the fundamental leg for the treatment of Foot Drop. The strengthening and stretching exercises that physical therapists have at their disposal are essential in the re-education of your muscles, as well as prevention of stiffness and gait improvement.[8] [9] Your physical therapist will work hand-in-hand with you to

---

[7] Xtern® by TurboMed™ Orthotics
https://turbomedorthotics.com/en/products/turbomed-xtern-external-ankle-foot-orthosis
[8] Foot Drop by Michael Walden August 2, 2019 on Sportsinjuryclinic.net website Pg. 2
[9] Foot Drop (Feet Muscle Weakness) Posted by Dr. Chris Pg. 4

maintain your range of motion in your knee and ankle. I have two words of wisdom where physical therapy and therapists are concerned: do your exercises and make your physical therapist your ally!

3. **Functional Electrical Stimulation** – your physical therapist places electrodes along the peroneal nerve of your affected leg and delivers a current to stimulate the nerve and thereby the muscle needed to lift the foot. These electrical bursts are usually timed to lift the foot during the "swing phase" of walking to prevent it from dropping or dragging.[10]

4. **Medication** – Primarily, this treatment focuses of the easement of pain and speed of healing. There are also medications that may be used for the treatment of underlying symptoms. The most common medications used would be:

---

[10] How to Keep Walking With MS-Related Foot Drop by Regina Boyle Wheeler Medically Reviewed by Farrokh Sohrabi, MD Reviewed: August 10, 2015 Pg. 5

- Tricyclic antidepressants and anticonvulsants may be used for pain.
- Application of diclofenac or capsaicin can also ease the pain.
- Narcotics like morphine are prescribed only in severe cases.
- Erythropoietin   [ə͵riTHrōˈpoiətn] treatment speeds up the recovery after nerve injury.[11]

5. **Surgery** – let me preface this section by saying this option is not for every case of Foot Drop. These are usually for cases with damaged or compressed nerves are directly responsible for the Foot Drop; in these instances, surgery might be able to decompress the nerve, or a nerve graft or transfer could be performed to repair it.[12] If the damage is permanent, your doctor might suggest surgery that fuses ankle or foot bones or a procedure that transfers a working tendon and attached muscle to a different part of the foot.[13]

---

[11] Foot Drop (Feet Muscle Weakness) Posted by Dr. Chris Pg. 4
[12] When Surgery Could Help Foot Drop Dr. Powers Foot and Ankle Website Pg. 1
[13] Foot Drop by Mayo Clinic Staff Mayo clinic website Pg. 2

This is a lot of information to digest! And, while it may seem overwhelming, remember this: you do not have to know it all; that is what your medical team is for. You need to make yourself familiar with your condition (because that is what Foot Drop is, a condition), and how to best facilitate the design of your exercise and physical therapy so you can get the most out of your effort. Also, you need to keep in contact with your MS support groups and find out how other fighters have coped with having to use some of these devices I have mentioned in past chapters, especially if and/or when you feel the devices compromise your feelings of independence. Remember – your journey will look the way you make it look. Make it your best, everyday!

References and Resources

1. *Foot Drop (Feet Muscle Weakness) Posted by Dr. Chris* https://www.healthhype.com/foot-drop-feet-muscle-weakness.html

2. *Drop Foot: symptoms, causes and treatments Written by Dr. Bob Baravarian, DPM, FACFAS Foot and Ankle Surgeon and Director of University Foot and Ankle Institute updated 8/11/2021*
https://www.footankleinstitute.com/conditions/drop-foot

3. *Xtern® by TurboMed™ Orthotics*
https://turbomedorthotics.com/en/products/turbomed-xtern-external-ankle-foot-orthosis

4. *Foot Drop by Michael Walden August 2, 2019 on Sportsinjuryclinic.net website*
https://www.sportsinjuryclinic.net/treatments-therapies/foot-biomechanics-gait-analysis/foot-drop

5. *How to Keep Walking With MS-Related Foot Drop by Regina Boyle Wheeler Medically Reviewed by Farrokh Sohrabi, MD Reviewed: August 10, 2015*
https://www.everydayhealth.com/multiple-sclerosis/symptoms/how-keep-walking-with-ms-related-foot-drop/

6. *When Surgery Could Help Foot Drop Dr. Powers Foot and Ankle Website*

https://bloomingtonpodiatrist.com/when-surgery-could-help-foot-drop/

7. *Foot Drop by Mayo Clinic Staff Mayo clinic website* https://www.mayoclinic.org/diseases-conditions/foot-drop/diagnosis-treatment/drc-20372633

8. *SaeboStep by Saebo* https://www.saebo.com/shop/saebostep/

9. *6 Stretches to Ease MS Symptoms by Lara DeSanto September 10, 2020* https://www.healthcentral.com/article/ms-best-stretches?ap=808&kw=multiple%20sclerosis%20symptoms%20treatment

10. *11 Exercises for Managing MS by Kristen Domonell, M.S., RYT Health Writer, Medical Reviewer Shaheen Lakhan, M.D. February 22, 2021* https://www.healthcentral.com/slideshow/best-exercises-ms

11. *Foot Drop: Symptoms and Causes by Mayo Clinic Staff* https://www.mayoclinic.org/diseases-

conditions/foot-drop/symptoms-causes/syc-20372628

12. *MS and Foot Drop by Devin Garlit May 4, 2016* https://multiplesclerosis.net/living-with-ms/foot-drop

Essay 7: MS & Bladder Control – This is NOT a Laughing Matter!

Imagine this: You are on your way to an appointment. Halfway there, your bladder, that you emptied before you left the house, tells you that it needs to be relieved. You figure you are almost to your destination, so you think of something else. You make it to your destination, and your bladder insists it be relieved – NOW!!! You take a deep breath (or several), clinch muscles you know are supposed to work, and proceed, telling your bladder that you will be going to the first Ladies' Room you come to. But your bladder is not satisfied and begins to spasm and tries to relieve itself in the middle of the long corridor with several onlookers.

You force your muscles to obey and tighten up; you reach the Ladies' Room, enter the stall, and just as you try to unbutton your pants – NIAGRA FALLS!!!! You try to minimize the damage, but you are now in full panic mode and have no control whatsoever. You have urinated on yourself, and you cry uncontrollably from the embarrassment, anger, and personal shame of not being able to control a bodily function that you have had a handle on for decades. You feel less than capable, less than human....

I don't have to imagine this scenario; I lived it. And to be honest, after going through this episode, I never wanted to leave my home again! In my mind, everyone I encountered could look at me and know what I had done. It was not until I began doing research into why my body was failing me due to my MS that I came across some remarkably interesting facts:

- Bladder (and bowel) problems occur commonly in MS.[1]

---

[1] Bladder and bowel issues from the MS International Federation website, Pg. 1

- At least 80% of MS patients are affected by bladder issues.[2]
- Up to 96 percent of patients who have MS for more than 10 years will experience urinary complications as a result of their condition.[3]

Why do bladder issues/problems affect the MS fighter to such a degree? ***Our signals are not being properly transmitted!!!*** Remember, MS causes lesions in the central nervous system (CNS); these lesions block or delay transmission of nerve signals that control the bladder and urinary sphincters.[4] When you have an overactive/spastic bladder (meaning you cannot hold a normal amount of urine), or a bladder that will not empty properly, the following symptoms, among others, can occur:

- Frequency and/or urgency of urination.
- Hesitancy in starting urination.
- Frequent nighttime urination (nocturia).

---

[2] Multiple sclerosis bladder control problems include incontinence and nocturia, Written by Emily Lunardo, Pg. 1

[3] An Overview of Bladder Dysfunction in MS by Julie Stachowiak, Ph.D., Pg. 1

[4] Bladder Problems from the National MS Society website. Pg. 2

- Incontinence (the inability to hold in urine).
- Inability to empty the bladder completely.[5]

I know many of you are saying, "I am NOT about to tell anyone, not even my doctor, that I cannot hold my water! It's too embarrassing!" Believe me, I totally understand; I was not willing to disclose this information either. But I had a choice to make - I could either tell my doctors what was going on with me and get appropriate treatment or be held hostage even further by my body and my condition/disease. I learned that attempting to ignore my condition could have led to:

- Permanent damage to the urinary tract.
- Urinary stones and UTI's (urinary tract infections).
- Localized skin infections.[6]
- **Urosepsis** - a type of sepsis that is caused by an infection in the urinary tract. It is a complication often caused by urinary tract

---

[5] 5 Bladder Problems from the National MS Society website. Pg. 2
[6] An Overview of Bladder Dysfunction in MS by Julie Stachowiak, Ph.D., Pgs. 2 & 3

infections that are not treated quickly or properly.[7]
- Isolation/restricted daily routines.
- Depression[8]
- Challenges with work, home, and social activities.
- Loss of independence, self-esteem, and confidence.[9]

Talking to your doctor will help you get your life back!!! He/she may prescribe medications for your issues. Your job is to be completely honest with your doctor. The best way to do this is to ask yourself some tough questions concerning your bladder issues. In an article entitled "Bladder Problems" from the National MS Society website, there is a PDF file with pertinent questions geared towards evaluating your bladder function.[10] This article also lists management and treatment options so you can be well-armored for your battle.

---

[7] Urosepsis: What to know about UTI complications, Medically reviewed by Xixi Luo, M.D. — Written by Jon Johnson on December 23, 2017, Pg. 1

[8] An Overview of Bladder Dysfunction in MS by Julie Stachowiak, Ph.D., Pg. 3

[9] Bladder Problems from the National MS Society website, Pg. 3

[10] Ibid, pg.3 (Questions to Ask Yourself about Your Bladder Health)

Now – let us talk about practical methods you need to employ once you and your doctor develop a treatment program. No treatment plan is going to work overnight, so you need to have a contingency plan in place for when you venture out in public:

- Plan frequent stops!
- Use and carry discreet protection, such as pads. These will give you confidence when you can't get to a bathroom.
- Wear easily removable clothes – such as trousers with an elastic waist or Velcro closures.
- Stash a change of clothes, underwear, pads, wipes, catheters, paper towels – whatever you need – in a tote bag or backpack that you bring with you.[11]

Bladder problems are nothing to laugh at; it's also nothing to hide from. Get over your embarrassment because you are not alone in this. Talk to your doctor because you need their help to make this situation better. And have your contingency plan(s) in place so you can get back

---

[11] Bladder Problems from the National MS Society website, Pg. 4

your independence and self-esteem. Life is so much better when you LIVE IT!!!

References and Resources

1. *Bladder and bowel issues Last Updated October27th, 2021*
https://www.msif.org/about-ms/symptoms-of-ms/bladder-and-bowel-issues/

2. *Multiple sclerosis bladder control problems include incontinence and nocturia*
https://www.belmarrahealth.com/multiple-sclerosis-bladder-control-problems-include-incontinence-and-nocturia

3. *An Overview of Bladder Dysfunction in MS*
https://www.verywellhealth.com/bladder-dysfunction-and-multiple-sclerosis-2440800

4. *Bladder Problems from the National MS Society website*
https://www.nationalmssociety.org/Symptoms-Diagnosis/MS-Symptoms/Bladder-Dysfunction

5. *Urosepsis: What to know about UTI complications*
https://www.medicalnewstoday.com/articles/320401

6. *Pelvic Floor Physical Therapy for MS: Help for Bladder, Bowel, and Sexual Function By Quinn Phillips, Medically Reviewed by Samuel Mackenzie, MD, PhD, Reviewed: November 6, 2020*
https://www.everydayhealth.com/multiple-sclerosis/pelvic-floor-physical-therapy-for-ms-help-for-bladder-bowel-and-sexual-function

Essay 8: It's Time to Talk About MS and Sexual Dysfunction

Let's keep it real – nobody wants to deal with sexual dysfunction! Why??? Because sexuality is part and parcel of who we are as people; it is one of the qualities by which we define ourselves. Being desired and feeling desirable is what makes the man/woman merry-go-round the incredible ride it is!!! So, when there is sexual dysfunction, you experience losses that are difficult to deal with, and your feelings about you and who you are affect you, your partner, and your relationship.

As I was doing my research on this topic (yes ma'am, yes sir, I have personal reasons for this topic!!!), I found out some rather interesting statistics concerning sexual dysfunction and MS:

- Sexual dysfunction is common among MS patients
- As many as 85% of men are affected
- Fifty percent to 75% of women are affected
- Seventy percent of people with MS have reported one or more sexual problems that interfered with sexual performance and/or pleasure much of the time.[1]

It makes sense; the feelings of sexual arousal start in the brain, down the spinal cord to the sexual organs. Well, MS causes the immune system to attack the myelin covering the spinal cord. This results in the formation of scars, or sclera, on the spinal cord, which causes delayed, missed, or confused signals to the body. The results look like:

Women –

- Loss of libido
- Vaginal dryness
- Difficulty achieving orgasm

---

[1] Sexual dysfunction written by the Editorial Team of the MultipleSclerosis.net website, January 29, 2013, Pg. 1

- Decreased sensation/painfully heightened sensation in the vaginal/clitoral area

Men –

- Loss of libido
- Erectile dysfunction
- Decreased sensation in the penis
- Inability or difficulty in reaching an orgasm[2] [3] [4] [5]

So, it makes sense that these messed up signals would be sent to our sexual organs. I know; it sounds good on paper, but in reality, it does not help!

Now that we have an idea of what we may be dealing with – HOW DO WE GET TO THE BOTTOM OF OUR DILEMMA? The first thing we have to do is be honest with ourselves and admit

---

[2] MS Sexual Problems: What you need to know from the Overcoming Multiple Sclerosis website, Pgs. 2 & 3

[3] Sexual dysfunction written by the Editorial Team of the MultipleSclerosis.net website, January 29, 2013, Pgs. 2 & 3

[4] Why MS Can Cause Sexual Dysfunction in Men — and What You Can Do About It, written by Erin Glace PT, MSPT, PRPC, BCB-PMD on September 21 2020, Pgs. 1 & 2

[5] Sexual Dysfunction in Multiple Sclerosis, the Cleveland Clinic website, Pgs. 1 & 2

there is a problem. This is not an easy admission by any means. Not being able to perform sexually with your partner is a devastating circumstance, and our first response is to internalize the pain and ignore the issue. That is neither healthy nor productive. The result of this inaction is going to be the loss of self-esteem, loss of self-confidence, anger, stress, and serious depression. You are also going to do a great deal of harm to your relationship by not being honest.

So, the second thing you have to do is HAVE A CONVERSATION WITH YOUR PARTNER! You are not in your relationship alone; your partner, spouse, or significant other is involved as well. You cannot hide this from them because, truth be told, they already know something has changed! They are not blind nor are they oblivious to the fact that your performance has significantly changed. They are stressed and angry because **you** are stressed and angry. More importantly, they are stressed because you do not trust them with the truth, and they are helpless to fix the issue. So have the hard conversation with your loved one!

The third thing is to TALK TO YOUR DOCTOR! Make no mistake - you are going to have feelings of embarrassment and shame; your bruised pride is going to play a large part, but you have the best resource readily available and at your disposal. Did you know that, according to a report by the National Multiple Sclerosis Society, 63% of us with MS have never talked about our sexual issues with our healthcare providers?[6] We ignore our greatest asset and source of information and assistance! If you need help in making the "talk" easier for you there is *The Multiple Sclerosis Intimacy and Sexuality Questionnaire (MSISQ-19).*[7] It is comprised of 19 questions to determine which of the three categories of sexual dysfunction you fall into:

- **Primary** – Refers to physiological impairment associated with lesions in the cortex and spinal cord which can lead to numbness or paresthesia (abnormal

---

[6] Why MS Can Cause Sexual Dysfunction in Men — and What You Can Do About It, written by Erin Glace PT, MSPT, PRPC, BCB-PMD on September 21 2020, Pg. 2

[7] The Multiple Sclerosis Intimacy and Sexuality Questionnaire (MSISQ-19), Sander AS, Foley FW, LaRocca NG, Zemon V.

burning or prickling of the skin) that directly affect the genitals; loss of libido; decreased vaginal lubrication in women; and difficulty initiating or maintaining an erection in men.

- **Secondary** – These are non-sexual physical changes such as fatigue, spasticity, pain, and bladder and bowel dysfunction.
- **Tertiary** - Psychosocial variables that can interfere with sexual performance or satisfaction, including changes in social roles, depression, demoralization, and interpersonal difficulties. [8]

I must put a warning here concerning getting help from some MS doctors for sexual dysfunction. According to a study conducted by G. Griswald (2003), a group of MS doctors were surveyed, and it was discovered that sexual dysfunction is not readily assessed. Here is the breakdown of the results:

---

[8] Sexual Dysfunction in Multiple Sclerosis, the Cleveland Clinic website, Pgs. 3 through 6

- 44% said they do not assess sexual dysfunction because of the limited time they have with patients.
- 15.3% said this issue is "outside their role."
- 12.5% said it was due to patient discomfort.
- 6.9% blamed lack of professional training or discomfort.
- 5.6% cited other priorities.
- 2.8% stated limited medical coverage so they (patients) cannot afford treatment.
- 2.8% claimed it was too intrusive for patients.[9]

While it has been 18 years since this study was published, you may run into one or more of these issues with your doctor. Press forward anyway – this is why they get paid "the Big Bucks!!!"

Fourth thing to do – FOCUS ON YOUR TREATMENT. Your doctor, based on whether you fall into the Primary, Secondary or Tertiary

---

[9] Sexual Dysfunction in Multiple Sclerosis, the Cleveland Clinic website, Pgs. 3 through 6

categories, can prescribe the appropriate treatment for you, or can refer you to a counselor who specializes in sexual dysfunction. They may also be able to provide you with educational material that will help you and your partner get through this together.

References and Resources

1. *Sexual dysfunction written by the Editorial Team of the MultipleSclerosis.net website, January 29, 2013*
https://multiplesclerosis.net/symptoms/sexual-dysfuncion

2. *MS Sexual Problems: What you need to know*
https://overcomingms.org/about-multiple-sclerosis/ms-symptoms/ms-sexual-problems

3. *Why MS Can Cause Sexual Dysfunction in Men — and What You Can Do About It*
https://www.healthline.com/health/multiple-sclerosis/why-ms-can-cause-sexual-dysfunction-in-men-and-what-you-can-do-about-it

4. *Sexual Dysfunction in Multiple Sclerosis from the Cleveland Clinic website* https://my.clevelandclinic.org/departments/neurological/depts/multiple-sclerosis/ms-approaches/sexual-dysfunction-ms

5. *The Multiple Sclerosis Intimacy and Sexuality Questionnaire (MSISQ-19), Reprinted with permission from Sander AS, Foley FW, LaRocca NG, Zemon V.*https://www.med-iq.com/files/noncme/material/pdfs/MSISQ-191.pdf

6. *Sexual Problems from the National Multiple Sclerosis website* https://www.nationalmssociety.org/Symptoms-Diagnosis/MS-Symptoms/Sexual-Dysfunction

Essay 9: MS Can (and DOES) Take A Toll on Our Mental Health

I ran across a post of an MS fighter that plain broke my heart:

Diagnosed 5 years ago: Primary Progressive.
PreDX: Athletic, near boundless energy and endurance
Now: Struggle to stay upright, tire easily
PreDX: Good dexterity, played saxophone, "Home Row" typing
Now: Difficulty grasping and holding things, SLOW typing.
PreDX: lifeguard, 10-12 hr. days at the pool and outside
Now: Temp over 80F/27C is debilitating
PreDX: Capable, independent, contributing member of society

Now: BARELY capable and independent. Fast becoming a drain on society and incapable of providing for myself.
Is there any reason for me to hang around for total disability and dependency? Having a hard time coming up with reasons, y'all. I'm not QUITE at the end of the rope but my hands are getting pretty tired.[1]

I felt a myriad of emotions after reading this post. The first was empathy as he and I have the same type of MS. The second was fear – fear that this could be me swimming in these same emotions down the line. The third emotion was urgency – the urgency to tell this person that, while life with MS is vastly different from what they were used to, life was still very much worth living and there was more than plenty of time before they got to the "end of their rope!!!"

After I thought long and hard about this individual and his plight, I decided to research the condition of depression as it relates to MS. I found some interesting facts:

---

[1] Facebook Group, Multiple Sclerosis (MS) Fitness & Exercise Motivation with Dom Thorpe

1. People with Multiple Sclerosis are 2 to 3 times more likely to become depressed than those without the condition.
2. Up to half of people with MS will experience depression at some point in their lives.[2]

But let us back up a bit and talk about what depression is. **Depression** is defined as

- *a mood disorder marked especially by sadness, inactivity, difficulty in thinking and concentration, a significant increase or decrease in appetite and time spent sleeping, feelings of dejection and hopelessness, and sometimes suicidal tendencies.*[3]

We must also understand why the MS fighter is far more susceptible to depression. We have talked about the lesions along the central nervous system (nerve damage) that are responsible for sending delayed/mixed/improper signals to the muscles; these signals can also be sent to the brain, which could cause people with MS to interpret feelings and situations in more

---

[2] Depression and MS: Ways to Care for Your Mental Health from the Healthline website, Pg. 1
[3] Merriam-Webster Online Dictionary

exacerbated ways. Not to mention that living with a chronic illness can cause anxiety and stress, and the drugs to treat MS (steroids and interferons) can cause depression as a side effect.[4] [5] Some other causes or symptoms of depression for the MS fighter can range from insomnia, fatigue, self-imposed isolation, loss of interest in everyday activities, feelings of guilt and worthlessness, loss/increased appetite, irritability, sadness, problems with thinking or concentration, and persistent thoughts of suicide.[6]

We must understand that depression is not controlled by willpower or determination and does not, in any way, indicate weakness of character. It is nothing to be ashamed of nor is it something that needs to be hidden.[7]

Now, before you jump off the deep end about being depressed, it is normal for people to experience being sad or "down in the dumps"

---

[4] Depression and MS: Ways to Care for Your Mental Health from the Healthline website, Pg. 1
[5] Multiple Sclerosis and Mental Health: 3 Common Challenges, Reviewed By: Meghan L. Beier, M.A., Ph.D., Pg. 3

[6] Depression from the National Multiple Sclerosis Society website, Pg. 3
[7] Ibid, pg. 1

from time to time. Even grieving is considered normal. Clinically a diagnosis of depression should be made by your doctor if your sadness has been continuous for two weeks or more. If this is what is going on with you, then absolutely take a closer look!

Ask yourself these questions:

- Do you always feel sad, hopeless, helpless, worthless, or empty?
- Are you more irritable than usual? Do you snap at the people around you?
- Have you lost interest in things you once loved to do? Does nothing you do seem to excite you?
- Do you feel extra tired or drained of energy?
- Do you have trouble sleeping, or sleep too much?
- Do you have difficulty concentrating or remembering?
- Do you notice strange aches and pains that you cannot connect to a physical cause?

- Have you noticed any changes in your appetite? Either eating too much or too little? [8]

Once you have spoken to your doctor or neurologist, they may decide to change your medication (as some therapies for MS cause depression). They may also have you speak with a counselor, psychologist, or a psychiatrist to develop strategies to help you better cope with your condition (preferably one who has experience working with MS patients).

There are also some other strategies you can utilize to cope with depression. Remember, it is just as important to take care of your emotional health as it is to take care of your physical health. Here are some things to try:

- Exercise daily.
- Reduce stress in your life and strive to manage inevitable stresses more calmly. Try breathing exercises and meditation.

---

[8] Depression and MS: Ways to Care for Your Mental Health from the Healthline website, Pg. 2

- Maintain your social networks. Call your friends. Join a support group. Spend time with family.
- Stay in touch with your medical team.
- Acknowledge your feelings. Get a notebook and write. Make a list of your stressors so you can stop thinking about them for a bit.
- Stay away from addictive substances such as alcohol.[9]

The one thing I love about researching information about MS is that there is a plethora of information and resources available to the MS fighter, so they do not have to fight alone. One such resource is the Depression and Multiple Sclerosis Brochure[10], available on the National Multiple Sclerosis Society website. Written by Sarah L. Minden, M.D., a psychiatrist at Brigham and Women's Hospital, this brochure talks about depression and MS in depth using language that is clearly understood by anyone reading it.

---

[9] Depression from the National Multiple Sclerosis Society website, Pg. 2
[10] Depression & Multiple Sclerosis Brochure BY SARAH MINDEN, M.D. © 2019

Additional resources are listed in the brochure as well.

Our emotional health is just as important as our physical health; truth be told, they go together, hand in hand. We must be prepared and equipped to care for them both or lose them both.

References and Resources:

1. *Facebook Group, Multiple Sclerosis (MS) Fitness & Exercise Motivation with Dom Thorpe*

2. *Depression and MS: Ways to Care for Your Mental Health*
https://www.healthline.com/health/ms/depression-and-ms

3. *Merriam-Webster Online Dictionary*
https://www.merriam-webster.com/dictionary/depression

4. *Multiple Sclerosis and Mental Health: 3 Common Challenges, Reviewed By: Meghan L. Beier, M.A., Ph.D.*
https://www.hopkinsmedicine.org/health/conditions-and-diseases/multiple-sclerosis-

ms/multiple-sclerosis-and-mental-health-3-
common-challenges

5. *Depression from the National Multiple Sclerosis Society website*
https://www.nationalmssociety.org/Symptoms-Diagnosis/MS-Symptoms/Depression

6. *Depression & Multiple Sclerosis Brochure Depression & Multiple Sclerosis Brochure BY SARAH MINDEN, M.D. © 2019*
https://www.nationalmssociety.org/NationalMS
Society/media/MSNationalFiles/Brochures/Broc
hure-Depression.pdf

7. 5 *Myths about MS and Depression, Medically Reviewed by Abbey Hughes, M.A., Ph.D.*
https://www.hopkinsmedicine.org/health/condi
tions-and-diseases/multiple-sclerosis-ms/5-
myths-about-multiple-sclerosis-and-depression

8.*National Crisis Hotline 1-800-273-TALK (8255) or text "ANSWER" to 839863*

Essay 10: What to Do When it Hits You All at Once

During the time around Mother's Day, I went through a couple of changes and had a few events go on in my life. I got my first COVID-19 vaccine shot, I had a Genicular Nerve Block performed on my knee due to consistent and chronic pain, and I was going through a depression that, as I now look back, has been with me for well over a year. All these factors led up to one thing – a massive meltdown!!! I had no energy nor the will to accomplish anything; I was drowning....

I had to push the pause button on my life for a moment and assess my situation and try, if possible, to produce alternate avenues for dealing with my overall state. So, here is what I saw:

- The COVID-19 vaccine: no real side effects, save the pain at the injection site. Not a factor in my current state.
- The Genicular Nerve Block: while the actual procedure only took 5 minutes, the general anesthesia stayed in my system for 24 hours or so. Could be a factor....
- The depression I had been feeling for the past 17 months; having to fight with myself about my current physical state, fighting with doctors about reassessing my condition, being diagnosed with MS, and trying to live my life with MS while not fully accepting my MS has taken a toll on me.
- I was in a state of grief: my dog/child of over 10 years passed away in January, and I had never really grieved my mother's death from over eight years ago. This Mother's Day I truly felt the absence of my mother and envied everyone that could still hold and speak to theirs. Lastly, I was grieving the losses I encountered from my MS (my loss of mobility, thereby leading to

my loss of independence). MAJOR FACTORS!!!

Now I see what is going on; I have had a major cave-in! I am emotionally exhausted. This is my truth. Now, I must decide what to do about it. There's Option #1: ignore what I am feeling and continue to go down this path. This is so not smart! If I can see the crash coming, the rational thing to do is to avoid crashing, thereby eliminating self-harm. Then there's Option #2: choose a different path, forge ahead with the same unresolved issues and eventually crash on that road. This is the inevitable outcome as the initial damage still hasn't been addressed. Now comes Option#3: pull over in a safe area, assess my damage, and call for assistance/help. Once the damage has been repaired, I can continue along whichever path I choose, knowing I am strong enough to continue.

I authored an article about a year or so ago entitled "I'm Tired Doesn't Mean I QUIT." Essentially the article says there is nothing wrong with taking a pause to regroup, reenergize and refresh. And that holds true for all people in all situations but especially for the MS fighter – recognize your need to rest and rejuvenate and act accordingly! Be it for an hour, a day, a month, whatever period of time you think you need. It will be okay, and it beats running yourself into the ground!!!

Section 2: Disease Modifying Therapies

Essay 11: Navigating Through the Medicinal Treatments

When I was first diagnosed with MS, I was not in shock, disbelief, or fear; I was relieved that I had finally received an accurate diagnosis. I now had a name for my nemesis, and a plan of attack. It was now time to arm myself with all the information I could about my disease and my medication so I could help in my treatment. What I found was there is a sea of information you can get bogged down in if you are not careful! And, if you try to dive in without guidance, YOU WILL DROWN!!!

Many people know there is a method to getting through the medicinal information madness, but for those who do not, let us go through the steps:

1. **<u>You get the diagnosis.</u>** Once your neurologist has done a detailed medical history, neurological exam, and a battery of tests (MRI's, spinal tap, blood tests), a proper and accurate diagnosis can be made as to which form of MS you have (Clinically Isolated Syndrome [CIS]/ Relapsing-Remitting MS [RRMS]/ Primary-Progressive MS [PPMS]/ Secondary-Progressive MS [SPMS]).[1] You and you neurologist will then discuss...

2. **<u>Treatment options.</u>** The one thing your neurologist is going to make clear to you, regardless of with type of MS you have been diagnosed with, MS at this point can only be controlled, not cured. With the exception of Primary Progressive MS, there are laundry lists of DMT'S (Disease Modification Therapies) for the remaining

---

[1] MS Medications by Joseph Bennington-Castro, Medically Reviewed by Samuel Mackenzie, MD, PhD Reviewed: May 3, 2020

forms of MS.[2] [3] These therapies may require you to take several medications at one time or consecutively. The one thing you must understand is that all medications, regardless of what they treat, have side effects; make sure you discuss these with your neurologist, but you should also take notes during your appointment (unless you can remember everything your neurologist says) and then...

3. **<u>DO YOUR OWN RESEARCH!</u>** Once you get the name(s) of your medication(s), look them up! We have so much information available to us now, thanks to Google, Bing, Firefox, and any other search engine you can think of to access the internet. Look up your medication for what it is approved to treat, as well as for the side effects. If there is any concern or objection you have to the medication's side effects –

4. **<u>Talk to your neurologist!</u>** Your neurologist needs to know if you are

---

2 DISEASE-MODIFYING THERAPIES FOR MS Brochure Updated July 2021
3 MS Medications by Joseph Bennington-Castro, Medically Reviewed by Samuel Mackenzie, MD, PhD Reviewed: May 3, 2020

comfortable with the course of action you are embarking on! Let's be honest; you are more likely to have a better result with your treatment if you have faith in the treatment. Your neurologist will not get mad if you voice your concerns (and if he/she does, you have the WRONG NEUROLOGIST!!!). Quiet as this is kept, all doctors appreciate patients that are participatory in their treatment. Also, as you proceed with your disease modifying treatment(s), keep your neurologist informed of how you are feeling while on the medications; if you experience any of the known side effects (or, you have a side effect that was not on the list), your neurologist needs to know so they can make the decision to change your medications.

5. <u>**Understand what your neurologist (or any doctor) truly is!**</u> Many people, me included, have had the wrong idea of what doctors are and what they are for. Yes, they are there to treat our illnesses and produce the medical plans of action, but we must stop seeing them as deities that are

infallible and cannot be questioned! That is unrealistic and it's an extreme amount of undue pressure to be harbored with. Instead, see your physician for what he/she is in truth: a wellspring of information from which you can draw from and/or add to. The medical profession is doing research on MS all the time and current information comes out as fast as they can get it published, but doctors do not have the time to read it all! If you find a treatment you find interesting and may want to try, email your neurologist. They may know about it, they may not, but you want to get their take on it, *always.* If your neurologist feels this treatment may be beneficial to you and will not cause any interaction with your prescribed therapies, he/she may approve it for you! Your job will then be to communicate with your doctor as to how the modification is going.

I hope this has been of some help to you. Remember – your MS looks the way you make it look!!!

<u>Resources and References:</u>

1. *MS Medications by Joseph Bennington-Castro, Medically Reviewed by Samuel Mackenzie, MD, PhD Reviewed: May 3, 2020* <u>https://www.everydayhealth.com/multiple-sclerosis/guide/medications/#side-effects%20for%20rrms</u>

2. *DISEASE-MODIFYING THERAPIES FOR MS Brochure Updated July 2021* <u>https://www.nationalmssociety.org/NationalMSSociety/media/MSNationalFiles/Brochures/Brochure-The-MS-Disease-Modifying-Medications.pdf</u>

3. *Medications* <u>https://www.nationalmssociety.org/Treating-MS/Medications</u>

4. *Drugs & Supplements: Ocrevus Reviewed: June 23, 2020*, <u>https://www.everydayhealth.com/drugs/ocrevus#sideeffects</u>

5. *MS Overview from the More to MS Website* https://www.moretoms.com/living-with-ms.html

6. *Statin Therapy Inhibits Remyelination in the Central Nervous System, American Journal Of Pathology, May 2009* https://www.researchgate.net/publication/24260411_Statin_Therapy_Inhibits_Remyelination_in_the_Central_Nervous_System

Section 3: Exercise

Essay 12: If You Want to Continue to Move, You MUST CONTINUE TO MOVE!!!

I have not always been on the best of terms with exercise. In truth, I have been through about four personal trainers during my adult dieting/fitness career, spent more than $15,000.00 to $20,000.00 dollars on trainers and gym memberships during that time period. I learned one undeniable truth about myself – I HATE EXERCISING!!! That was my detrimental short-term mentality. What I should have learned was that exercise is a long-term lifestyle to which you must commit. The more consistent you are with an exercise regiment, the healthier you tend to be in the long run.

Now that I have Multiple Sclerosis, this lesson is slapping me in the face every single day! Why? Because now, like it or not, I must exercise every single day, because exercising makes my mobility easier, it makes my mobility possible! The more I exercise, the greater amount of strength I have to get through my day. On the days I make the mistake of choosing NOT to engage in exercise, I feel lethargic, fatigued, and I find all tasks insurmountable. So, every morning, I spend a minimum of 15 minutes doing my stretching exercises for my benefit.

But how do you select an exercise plan that is right for you? MS creates a unique set of physical limitations that must always be a primary concern. So where do you start?

- **<u>Talk to your neurologist or primary care physician.</u>** This should be your first line of information before you begin your exercise journey! You need to know where you are physically *at this moment,* not where you were prior to diagnosis. Your neurologist may suggest that you start physical therapy in order to facilitate your movement.

- **<u>Do your research!</u>** If you feel confident enough to exercise on your own, or you want to supplement your physical therapy, Google, Bing, Firefox, and all search engines can give you the resources for exercises that are best suited to MS. For example, yoga, aqua exercising, stretching, weight training, aerobic exercising (this includes dancing), Pilates, and Tai Chi are among the top forms of exercises recommended for MS[1]. There are also other resources, such as the Multiple Sclerosis Foundation[2], not to mention there are books on this subject (probably the most user-friendly book is Multiple Sclerosis for Dummies by Rosalind Kalb, Barbara Giesser, and Kathleen Costello[3]).
- **<u>Look into a personal trainer.</u>** Admittedly, this option can get to be a bit expensive if you are not careful. Also, you must, for your own safety, find a trainer

---

[1] Exercise, from the National multiple Sclerosis Society website, Pgs. 3 & 4
[2] Multiple Sclerosis Foundation (website)
[3] Multiple Sclerosis for Dummies: 2nd Edition Paperback by Rosalind Kalb (Author) Barbara Giesser, and Kathleen Costello – April 13, 2012

who is versed in Multiple Sclerosis so that no harm is done to you in the name of assisting you. Not all trainers are going to be mindful of your limitations. My personal choice was the MS Warriors Programme©[4]. This program was designed by Dom Thorpe, a fitness trainer who has first-hand knowledge and experience dealing with MS clients and breaks the exercises into levels – mobile, walks with assistance, wheelchair/limited mobility. He is affordable, too....

- **<u>COMMIT, COMMIT, COMMIT TO YOUR CHOICE!!!</u>** Regardless of your chosen method of exercise, none of these options will work if you are not committed to making them work!!! Remember, your MS is going to look the way YOU MAKE IT LOOK. So, if you want to continue to move, you must continue to move. MS comes with a myriad of symptoms, the most dangerous (in my opinion) being impaired balance, coordination, and mobility.

---

[4] MS Warrior Programme by Dom Thorpe - website

Your quality of life (QOL) is entirely in your hands. Get up and move!!!

References and Resources:

1. *Exercise, from the National multiple Sclerosis Society* https://www.nationalmssociety.org/Living-Well-With-MS/Diet-Exercise-Healthy-Behaviors/Exercise

2. *Multiple Sclerosis Foundation* https://msfocus.org/

3. *Multiple Sclerosis for Dummies: 2nd Edition Paperback by Rosalind Kalb (Author) Barbara Giesser, and Kathleen Costello – April 13, 2012* https://www.amazon.com/Multiple-Sclerosis-Dummies-Rosalind-Kalb/dp/1118175875

4. *MS Warrior Programme* https://dt-training.co.uk/ms-warrior-programme/

5. *Benefits of Tai Chi for Multiple Sclerosis by Lisa Emrich Patient Advocate May 25, 2017* https://www.healthcentral.com/article/benefits-of-tai-chi-for-multiple-sclerosis

6*. HOW HIP OPENING YOGA POSES CAN IMPROVE YOUR DAY JESSE SAGE May 31, 2020* https://yogapose.com/articles/how-hip-opening-yoga-poses-can-improve-your-day

7*. 6 Simple Stretches to Do Every Morning and Night Advil + RealSimple* https://www.realsimple.com/featured/StriveSimpleStretchesToDoEveryMorningAndNight

8*. 10 Best Exercises to Boost Wellness When You Have Multiple Sclerosis By Beth W. Orenstein Medically Reviewed by Jason Paul Chua, MD, PhD Reviewed: May 26, 2021* https://www.dummies.com/health/diseases/exercise-options-for-multiple-sclerosis-patients

9*. Multiple Sclerosis: 30-day exercise program Written by the Healthline Editorial Team on August 20, 2018* https://www.healthline.com/health/multiple-sclerosis/exercise-challenge#1

10*. MS Exercises for Better Balance and Coordination Medically reviewed by Daniel Bubnis, M.S., NASM-CPT, NASE Level II-CSS, Fitness Written by Kimberly Holland — Updated on June 25, 2020* https://www.healthline.com/health/multiple-sclerosis/exercises-balance-coordination#weight-training

11. *MS Exercises for Better Balance and Coordination Medically reviewed by Daniel Bubnis, M.S., NASM-CPT, NASE Level II-CSS, Fitness Written by Kimberly Holland — Updated on June 25, 2020* https://www.healthline.com/health/multiple-sclerosis/exercises-balance-coordination#exercises-for-balance

Essay 13: "No Pain, No Gain" Will Do More Harm than Good!

Recently in a Facebook group I follow for MS warriors (Multiple Sclerosis {MS} Fitness & Exercise Motivation with Dom Thorpe[1]), there were several posts from members talking about how they were really pushing themselves to the point of pain and exhaustion. And the one catch phrase they all used was, "No pain, no gain, right?" I do not think any of these members were ready for the onslaught of negative responses they were given for this mindset....

I had to really think about that before I answered. They really did not say anything

---

[1] Multiple Sclerosis {MS} Fitness & Exercise Motivation with Dom Thorpe, Facebook

wrong, in the sense that we have been PROGRAMMED to adopt this mindset! Think about it; sport athletics, weight loss, academics – we hear this phrase ad nauseum, "NO PAIN, NO GAIN!!! If you want more, you have to give more! Dig 'til it hurts, then dig deeper! That's how winners are made!!!" Well, that is true, provided you are of average strength and health levels. Having MS takes us out of this 'no pain no gain' realm and forces us into the 'do a little, rest a little' category.

What do I mean by that? It's like this; our central nervous systems now have frays in the wiring, causing us to have short circuits, if you will, in the messages from our brains to our muscles. For us to maintain the same (or even close to the same) control over our muscle movements takes far more energy than ever before! This causes us to tire faster and crash harder than the "normal" individual. So, for our protection and our progression, we must abandon "no pain, no gain" for "do a little, rest a little."

Now, I am sure that there are those who would disagree with me, and that is fine. But my point of view has validity from the National MS

Society, who published the blog article entitled "Exercise." Here are their tips for a successful workout:

- Stay hydrated - cold water will help keep your body temperature low.
- Exercise in a cool room and if outside, exercise at cooler times during the day.
- Remember to stretch afterward.
- *No pain no gain should not be your mantra!!!*
- Start low and go slow.
- Consult a medical professional before starting a new exercise routine.
- Prioritize safety to reduce risk of injury.[2]

The purpose of exercise for us is to regain and/or retain our levels of mobility; too much too fast will derail our progress.

It is also important with your exercise to set manageable goals for yourself. To do this, you do not look at what you used to do; that no longer applies. Talk to your doctors; he/she will be more than happy to assist you in devising a fitness plan, or they may set you up with

---

[2] Exercise, from the National Multiple Sclerosis Society website, Pg. 3

physical therapy.[3] After a time, your PT can suggest additional exercises for you to do on your own.

To help you understand your new "exercise normal," make it a cogent point to connect yourself to as many MS resources as you can! Go to Facebook[4], the Above MS website[5], the National MS Society[6], even the Mayo Clinic website[7]. These resources are invaluable to you and will provide you with points of reference for your exercise goals and beyond. You are not alone in this!!!

Please keep this in mind: always, ALWAYS keep your goals realistic and manageable for who and where you are *right now.* Remember, MS fighters fatigue faster and exercise that's too aggressive for your current abilities will bring on fatigue, injury, and exacerbate your symptoms.[8] What you used to do is no longer your concern; focus on your here and now. Take pride in your

---

[3] Exercise and multiple sclerosis from the Mayo Clinic website, Pg.1
[4] Facebook - https://www.facebook.com
[5] The Above MS Website https://www.abovems.com/
[6] National MS Society | Official Site https://secure.nationalmssociety.org/
[7] Mayo Clinic Website https://www.mayoclinic.org
[8] Exercise and multiple sclerosis from the Mayo Clinic website, Pg.1

accomplishments and rejoice in your current successes.

I have one last thing to add: never forget that you, regardless of your MS diagnosis, *are still you!!!* Everything that propelled you to be capable at everything you did prior to your MS diagnosis is still within you, waiting for you to tap into it! I'd be lying if I said there won't be some setbacks, but if you let go of the "no pain, no gain" mindset, you are assured far more successes than setbacks. Set yourself up for success and "do a little, rest a little." YOU GOT THIS!!!

References and Resources

1. Multiple Sclerosis {MS} Fitness & Exercise Motivation with Dom Thorpe, Facebook
https://www.facebook.com/groups/156982148287076

2. *Exercise, from the National Multiple Sclerosis Society website*
https://www.nationalmssociety.org/Living-Well-

With-MS/Diet-Exercise-Healthy-
Behaviors/Exercise

3. *Exercise and Multiple Sclerosis from the
Mayo Clinic website*
https://www.mayoclinic.org/diseases-
conditions/multiple-sclerosis/expert-
answers/exercise-and-multiple-sclerosis/faq-
20094108

4. *Facebook* - https://www.facebook.com

5. *The Above MS Website*
https://www.abovems.com/

6. *National MS Society | Official Site*
https://secure.nationalmssociety.org

7. *Mayo Clinic Website*
https://www.mayoclinic.org

8. *Celebrating life with MS*
https://www.abovems.com/en_us/home/ms-
wellness/mental-emotional-health/celebrating-
life-with-ms.html

9. *4 tips on aging with MS*

https://www.abovems.com/en_us/home/ms-wellness/exercise-fitness/healthy-aging-ms.html

10. *Exercise from the National MS Society website*
https://www.nationalmssociety.org/Living-Well-With-MS/Diet-Exercise-Healthy-Behaviors/Exercise

11. *Exercise Training Guidelines for Multiple Sclerosis, Stroke, and Parkinson Disease: Rapid Review and Synthesis*
https://pubmed.ncbi.nlm.nih.gov/30844920/

12. *Effects of exercise training on fitness, mobility, fatigue, and health-related quality of life among adults with multiple sclerosis: a systematic review to inform guideline development*
https://pubmed.ncbi.nlm.nih.gov/23669008/

Section 4: Diet

Essay 14: Food and MS - Another Trip Down the "Confusion Rabbit Hole!!!"

I am a Foodie; I love food! My favorite store is the grocery store! For me, there is nothing more exciting and exhilarating than walking through the colorful produce aisles, taking in the seafood/meat/chicken selections, and imagining the meals I could prepare and how they would look, smell, and taste!!! I can just see the expressions of joy and amazement on the faces of my friends and family as they take their first bites, and I could imagine their looks of total satisfaction as they reached their climactic culinary orgasm! Yes, tasty food does that for me!!!

I am also a career dieter…. I have, over the years, collected diet books, tried insane crash diets, and used about every diet remedy sold over the counter. My situation has always been this: I discover I am close to being clinically obese (meaning, I am almost 30 pounds over my clinical ideal weight), go on a crash diet to lose 30-35 pounds, maintain it for about 6 months, then rediscover food with a vengeance!!! The result was that I not only gained back the weight I lost, but my weight also comes back with about 15 of its wayward cousins!!!

When I was diagnosed with my Multiple Sclerosis, I was trying to get my weight under control because I was substantially unhealthy. I talked to my doctors, did my research, and consulted my personal library for direction and guidance. Do you know what I got? I got TOTALLY CONFUSED, that's what I got!!! Just as there are as many causes for MS as there are people with MS (practically), there are loads of ideas concerning diet and nutrition for MS. One article I read advocated eating oatmeal as a healthy grain in the beginning but denounced the use of oats by the end of the article (needless to say, that reference has NOT been used in the writing of this article). Some articles say that tomatoes and peppers should not be used in the MS diet plan, but so many of the recipes contain the very food items MS fighters are supposed to avoid. Like I said, it's confusing.

I was able to find five diet theories that seem to be the most popular for easing and/or controlling MS symptoms: Paleo, Mediterranean, Swank, Wahl, and Gluten-Free. Let us look at each one:

- **Paleo.** These plans favor lean meats, fish, vegetables, fruits, nuts, and berries and calls for the elimination of processed foods, grains, most dairy products, and refined sugars. The idea is that the body can process the acceptable ancient staples better than the more modern items. Additionally, this diet calls for the intake of game meats (bison, elk, venison, rabbit); this would make up close to 30 to 35 percent of your daily caloric intake. The research on paleo diets and MS is minimal at best.[1] [2]

- **Mediterranean Diet.** This traditional diet is considered the healthiest in the world. You will eat lots of fish, whole grains, fruits, veggies, legumes (edible seeds grown in a pod), and olive oil. It should be noted that this diet is not specific to MS and there is no research on how this diet affects MS. This diet is considered to be good for you in general.[3]

- **The Swank Diet.** Created by Dr Roy L. Swank, this diet is exceptionally low in saturated fat (maximum 15 grams/day). It also calls for eliminating processed foods that contain fat and hydrogenated oils. The emphasis is on whole grains, very lean proteins (skinless white meat poultry and white fish), fruits, vegetables, and whole grains. There is NO RED MEAT for the first

---

[1] Does Your Diet Affect Your MS? by Melinda Wenner Moyer, Medically Reviewed by Brunilda Nazario, MD, March 5, 2020, Pg. 2

[2] What to Know About MS and Diet: Wahls, Swank, Paleo, and Gluten-Free by Sara Lindberg, Medically Reviewed by Carissa Stephens, R.N., CCRN, CPN, Updated January 25, 2019, Pgs. 2 & 3

[3] Does Your Diet Affect Your MS? by Melinda Wenner Moyer, Medically Reviewed by Brunilda Nazario, MD, Updated March 5, 2020, Pg. 2

year of this diet, and only three ounces of red meat per week after the first year.[4]

- **The Wahls Protocol for MS.** Created by Terry Wahls, MD, an MS fighter herself, this paleo-like diet focuses on the role food plays in treating MS. The difference between this protocol and paleo is there is a greater emphasis on the consumption of vegetables to meet the body's optimal need for nutrition through food. This protocol calls for more deeply pigmented fruits and berries, green vegetables, and more sulfur-rich vegetables, such as mushrooms and asparagus.[5]
- **Gluten-Free Diet.** Because gluten causes inflammation in the body, there are those that hold with the belief that a gluten-free diet will eliminate this particular source of inflammation and decrease the symptoms of MS. There is no research, however, that supports this theory. But, if you have an

---

[4] What to Know About MS and Diet: Wahls, Swank, Paleo, and Gluten-Free by Sara Lindberg, Medically Reviewed by Carissa Stephens, R.N., CCRN, CPN, Updated January 25, 2019, Pgs. 4 & 5
[5] IBID., Pg. 4

allergy to gluten or suffer from celiac disease, this is the diet for you. A word of warning: this is the MOST RESTRICTIVE of all the diets![6] [7]

So, what is the right way to go??? You go back to what makes sense – you make your MS diet look the way you want it to look!!! I went about this using another tactic – I looked at foods I was told to avoid and worked from there. I eliminated red meat (good-bye steaks and pork chops), traded cow's milk for almond milk, kept cheese consumption to a minimum (I am not able to eat low-fat cheese just yet). I do not eat eggs anymore, I do one cup of caffeine a day: no sweets, cereal, breads, or grains. No fast foods, white potatoes, or pasta. I also watch my portions on the foods I can eat.

I also had to completely change my way of thinking about my new plan; this is not a short-term, quick fix for a couple of months. This is my new lifestyle, a permanent culinary adoption.

---

[6] What to Know About MS and Diet: Wahls, Swank, Paleo, and Gluten-Free by Sara Lindberg, Medically Reviewed by Carissa Stephens, R.N., CCRN, CPN, Updated January 25, 2019, Pgs. 4 & 5

[7] Does Your Diet Affect Your MS? by Melinda Wenner Moyer, Medically Reviewed by Brunilda Nazario, MD, Updated March 5, 2020, Pgs. 1 & 2

I cannot afford to keep my old, ineffective way of thinking about food and diet – NO MS FIGHTER CAN!!! Our objective, our goal, is to live a long and happy life with minimized MS symptoms. We can do this; we've got this!!!

References and Resources

1. *Does Your Diet Affect Your MS? by Melinda Wenner Moyer, Medically Reviewed by Brunilda Nazario, MD, Updated March 5, 2020* https://www.webmd.com/multiple-sclerosis/rrms-20/does-diet-affect-ms

2. *What to Know About MS and Diet: Wahls, Swank, Paleo, and Gluten-Free by Sara Lindberg, Medically Reviewed by Carissa Stephens, R.N., CCRN, CPN, Updated January 25, 2019* https://www.healthline.com/health/overview-diets-for-multiple-sclerosis

3. *The Best and Worst Foods for Multiple Sclerosis* https://www.ihealthself.com/food-and-nutrition/the-best-and-worst-foods-for-multiple-sclerosis

4. *Top Foods Multiple Sclerosis Patients Must Avoid*
https://www.brainfuel.online/lifestyle/top-foods-multiple-sclerosis-patients-must-avoid

5. *Food Groups to Avoid While Managing MS*
https://www.urbanious.com/health/food-groups-to-avoid-while-managing-ms

6. *6 Beneficial Foods for Multiple Sclerosis Patients*
https://www.healthconditions.net/health/6-beneficial-foods-for-multiple-sclerosis-patients

7. *5 Foods to Avoid for Multiple Sclerosis*
https://www.popnewsupdate.com/health/5-foods-that-can-aggravate-multiple-sclerosis-symptoms

8. *Foods to Avoid for Multiple Sclerosis*
https://www.wellnessfueled.com/diet/foods-to-avoid-for-multiple-sclerosis

Essay 15: Food and MS - Making the Best of What You Can Eat!

In the previous chapter, we talked about creating a diet plan based on foods you must avoid. Let's approach this from another angle: let us look on the positive side and create our new diet plan based on what we CAN EAT!!!

1. **We can eat FISH/SEAFOOD!** Oh, my God!!! What a plethora of varieties and choices open to you!!! Shellfish (shrimp, scallops, crab, lobster), salmon, cod, herring, mahi-mahi, rainbow trout, perch, mackerel – the list is long and succulent!!! And the recipes available for meal preparation make fish and seafood a treasure trove of possibilities!!! You do

have to exercise caution here and avoid fish selections that are (1) high in mercury content and (2) low in omega-3 oils.[1]

2. **Chicken and Turkey.** Yes, we all know that chicken and turkey are the basic staples in every diet known to modern man, but here is the good news: there are more recipes for these two items than any other food, hands down. You may not be able to batter and fry it, but you can prepare chicken it so many other ways! Take your pick – broiled, baked, grilled, boiled, pan-seared. You have so many options!

3. **Vegetables and Produce.** This is where you can let your imagination and courage take flight! Sure, you can stick to your tried-and-true staples but try expanding your horizons beyond what you are used to! Create a stir fry using Bok choy, broccoli, bean sprouts, spring onions, carrots, peppers, fresh ginger, and your choice of chicken or shellfish. If you are not sure how a vegetable should be prepared,

---

[1] Best and Worst Fish for Your Health (slideshow) on the Nourish by WebMD website

use Google, Bing, or any search engine of your choice. There is a recipe for whatever you choose to cook. Let your imagination run free!

4. **FRUIT!!!** You have no restrictions in this arena but watch out for excessive natural sugar overload! You can eat fruit!!! Au naturelle or in a smoothie, fruit is acceptable. Become adventurous here as well; pick samples of fruit you have never eaten and see if you like it. (You are only going to pick one as a sample, so you are not wasting a great deal of money! But, if you learn something new about yourself, was it really a waste?)

5. **Nuts.** This food is high in healthy fat, they taste great, there is a large variety, and they're accessible on the go! Between pecans, almonds, cashews, walnuts, and your Spanish and/or blanched peanuts, you have snacking made! Just watch out for the salted versions of these items as the salt will tend to make you retain water....

The right foods are essential for our fight against MS. You must consume three balanced meals every day, not to mention at least two between-meal snacks for optimal health. You can have a whole new culinary experience within the so-called limitations to your new eating lifestyle. Dive right in and have a blast!!!

Resources and References:

1. *Best and Worst Fish for Your Health (slideshow)* https://www.webmd.com/diet/ss/slideshow-best-worst-fish

2. *12 Best Types of Fish to Eat Medically reviewed by Natalie Olsen, R.D., L.D., ACSM EP-C — Written by Nicole Bowling, CPT — Updated on August 19, 2020* https://www.healthline.com/health/food-nutrition/11-best-fish-to-eat

3. *Jennie·O® Turkey website* https://www.jennieo.com/products/

4. *Butterball® Turkey website*
https://www.butterball.com/products

5. *Applegate Naturals® Turkey Bacon*
https://www.applegate.com/products/natural-
turkey-bacon

6. *6 Beneficial Foods for Multiple Sclerosis
Patients*
https://www.healthconditions.net/health/6-
beneficial-foods-for-multiple-sclerosis-patients

7. *Dr. Perricone's No. 7 Superfood: Hot
Peppers Published 07/15/2005*
https://www.oprah.com/health/hot-peppers-dr-
perricones-superfood-no-7-superfood/all

8. *43 Low Carb Vegetables* (Printable Chart!)
https://www.thelittlepine.com/low-carb-
vegetables/

9. *10 Low-Fat Cheeses You Can Eat When
You're Losing Weight by Emily Shiffer January
17, 2020* https://www.eatthis.com/low-fat-
cheese

10. *The 9 Healthiest Types of Cheese Written by Lizzie Streit, MS, RDN, LD on March 4, 2019* https://www.healthline.com/nutrition/healthiest -cheese

Section 5:
Caregivers, Family, & Friends

Essay 16: Caregivers - Our Saving Grace and Closest Aggravation

There will be no references in this essay; I just need to talk and try to make sense of what I am currently going through. Carl, my husband, my caregiver, is a good man and I consider myself very blessed to have him. My reality is that, at this stage of my MS fight, I rely on him more than ever before. It pains and physically distresses me to drive long distances, so he drives me to all my doctors' appointments, picks up the groceries I order, and he picks up my prescriptions on his way home from work in order to ease my burden. He even, at times, will help with the cooking or will pick up dinner when he sees I cannot function around the house and kitchen. I have no complaints in this arena.

BUT…. The other day, while I was preparing dinner, I started to feel fatigued, and my pain was increasing by leaps and bounds. My husband comes up from the basement, sees my condition, and asked me if I wanted him to take over. I was honestly relieved that he asked, and then… it happened. Just as I was about to say "Yes, I do! Thank you," my husband uttered two words that sent my mind reeling! He said: "LAST CHANCE." I gave no argument at that time only because I was in too much pain to give him the cussing-out I felt his statement deserved. I sat down and let him finish preparing dinner.

The next day, as we were driving to one of my many doctor's appointments, I asked him, "I've got to ask you – what did you mean by 'last chance?'"

"Huh?" says he.

"When you asked me last night if I wanted you to finish the dinner, you said 'last chance.' What did you mean by that?" Now, I am ready for the fight…

"I said that?"

"Yes."

"Oh, baby, I don't remember that."

"Why not?"

"Because I was just talking; it didn't mean anything."

I looked at my husband; either he was telling the truth, or he was really doing his best to nullify the impending discussion by feigning denial. Either way, I had to conserve my energy for walking through the medical building, so I let it go at that moment. What I could not let go of was the multitude of feelings those two words brought on: specifically, confusion, sadness, and RAGE.

Words are powerful; more powerful, I believe, than physicality. Used in the right way, words can be nurturing and solidify any relationship. However, when those same words are used in an off-hand, cavalier manner, they can cut deeper than any knife and the damage can be lifelong. Speaking for myself, I am acutely aware of what is said to me during my bouts of fatigue and pain. During these bouts, I am not up for a whole lot of off-the-cuff shade and drama!

Please do not think I am unaware of the added stress and strain my husband has had placed on his shoulders; my MS has affected him on many levels. And I do not discount the magnificent effort he expends being my caregiver; having cared for my mother during her fight with cancer, I know it is a lot of added responsibility to shoulder. But, while I am aware of the added burden my MS has added to our marital potluck, the one thing that has not sunk in for my husband is that what he is dealing with, though impactful, is residual. He does not suffer from any DIRECT SYMPTOMOLOGY OF MS. Saying something belittling and demeaning to your loved one, EVEN IN JEST, is not deserved.

While I am writing this to vent (and gripe), I am also writing this for our caregivers. Make no mistake – WE LOVE YOU SO MUCH!!! We know that we could not make it without your love and support, and it means more than you know to us that you are here with us and for us. We do not want you to NOT enjoy our lives together, but we could all just watch how we say what we want and need to say. Keeping things honest, we MS fighters may get a bit full of ourselves at times and let some nonsense fly out of our mouths too (we ain't always innocent victims) …

Essay 17: The MS Conversation - The Do's and Don'ts for Friends and Family

With the Spring weather slowly coming in, and the COVID 19 vaccine becoming available to all people, there are going to be family events in the future for me. Not to mention events with friends; the most prominent event coming up for me is going to be my 40-year high school reunion. And while I am looking forward to reconnecting with these friends, I am not looking forward to well-meaning (and some not-so-well-meaning) friends' uninformed and/or insensitive inquiries.

Don't get me wrong, most people do not mean to be insensitive, but because MS is not a disease that it widely spoken of, a lot of people have no idea what you are going through or what they should or should not say. To that end, let's look at some statements that could be made and how they could be said more tactfully and sensitively:

1. **How did you get MS? What did you do to get it?** No one with MS can tell you how they got it, just as no one can tell you how they got certain types of cancer or rheumatoid arthritis. MS is an autoimmune disease that can affect any gender, race, ethnicity, at any given time, and under a myriad of circumstances. A better way to ask would be: *"I do not know much about MS, could you educate me on what MS is? What is an autoimmune disease?"*[1] [2]

2. **You do not LOOK SICK.** I bought an MS t-shirt that reads: "I don't look sick? You don't look STUPID. Looks can be

---

[1] 11 Things You Should Never Say to Someone with MS Medically reviewed by the Healthline Medical Network — Written by Ann Pietrangelo — Updated on March 16, 2016 Pgs. 2-12

[2] MS & Things People Should NOT Say Bb Ashley Ringstaff June 25, 2013 Pgs. 2 & 3

deceiving...." You can't see the damage MS does to my spinal cord and brain; you will see some symptoms resulting from my MS. Change that to: _"You look great! So, how are you feeling?"_[3] [4]

3. **You should try this vitamin, that supplement and/or herb.** People try to help by telling you about what somebody's brother's uncle's cousin did and now they no longer have MS. At this point there is no medicine, herb or supplement that cures Multiple Sclerosis so, unless you hold a medical degree, please do not prescribe medications. Just say: _"Listen, if you feel like talking about it, I'd like to know how you are treating your MS."_[5]

4. **Why are you dragging your foot?** First, let me thank you for bringing so much unnecessary and unwanted attention to me and my current physical deficit by asking that question (and so loudly, too!). Let's

---

[3]   11 Things You Should Never Say to Someone with MS Medically reviewed by the Healthline Medical Network — Written by Ann Pietrangelo — Updated on March 16, 2016 Pgs. 2-12

[4]   MS & Things People Should NOT Say Bb Ashley Ringstaff June 25, 2013 Pgs. 2 & 3

[5] Ibid.

just say that there are rules of manners and etiquette that make that question rude and off-limits and should not be asked – EVER. [6]

5. **I know exactly how you feel – TRUST ME!** While I understand that most people see this as being empathetic and caring, it is in fact dismissive and insulting. What you have done in this statement is let me know that you have no interest in what I am telling you and you want the conversation to end. Sometimes we need to vent; you need to use three words: *"I believe you."*[7]

6. **I don't understand why you're tired all the time.** Here's the thing: because MS causes our central nervous systems to send mixed/wrong/delayed signals to our muscles, it takes far more physical and mental strength to get our everyday tasks accomplished than "normal" people. The MS fatigue is like nothing you have experienced, and the recovery time can be

---

[6] 11 Things You Should Never Say to Someone with MS Medically reviewed by the Healthline Medical Network — Written by Ann Pietrangelo — Updated on March 16, 2016 Pgs. 2-12
[7] Ibid.

lengthy. Here is an alternative to this statement: _"Don't worry about having to cancel, we'll reschedule when you're feeling better. This is not a problem."_ [8]

7. **Stop using MS as an excuse/crutch; you can't feel like that all the time!** This is just the most insensitive, hurtful, presumptuous thing you can say – barre none!!! This is when you fall back to the old adage: "If you can't say something nice, don't say anything at all!!!"[9] [10]

These are my top pet peeve statements concerning MS, but there are articles covering a multitude more of statements like these. Statements like:

- Maybe you should just try harder
- If you are in remission, why are you still on meds?
- Why do you keep forgetting things?

---

[8] MS & Things People Should NOT Say Bb Ashley Ringstaff June 25, 2013 Pgs. 2 & 3

[9] 11 Things You Should Never Say to Someone with MS Medically reviewed by the Healthline Medical Network — Written by Ann Pietrangelo — Updated on March 16, 2016 Pgs. 2-12

[10] MS & Things People Should NOT Say Bb Ashley Ringstaff June 25, 2013 Pgs. 2 & 3

- Are you contagious?
- I heard a vaccine caused MS.
- Maybe you should exercise more....
- If the heat bothers you, don't be in it...or move.
- It really can't be that bad.
- Are you sure it is MS? How can the doctors be so sure?[11] [12]

In short, we MS fighters know that, in the final analysis, our family and friends want the best for us, and they love us deeply. But it is all in the presentation of your statements and questions that will make the difference between a loving, caring conversation or having us give the standard "I'm fine" because we are not sure of the emotional temperature of the room.

Try statements and questions like these:

- How are you doing? (NOTE: be prepared to listen without judgement or interruption)

---

[11] Things people say to a person with multiple sclerosis...and shouldn't by Penelope Conway November 3, 2020
[12] Supporting Someone Who has MS from the MS Society website Pgs. 3 & 4

- How can I help? (NOTE: be honest about what help you can provide and say "NO" when you cannot give what is needed.)
- Ask your friend where to get information about MS so you can have a better understanding of the disease and they do not have to constantly explain MS to you.
- Say "I'm here for you." Continue to reach out.
- Just hang out. Make sure your friendship is about more than the MS and you helping. Have lunch, have a spa day, go shopping (provided your fighter will have access to an electric cart. That is essential!!!)
- Statements like "I am here for you," "I care about you," and "You can always lean on me" mean the world to MS fighters. It never hurts to hear that you are loved.[13] [14]

This is by no means a rebuff to friends and family. On the contrary, we need the people that

---

[13] What People SHOULD Say to Someone Living with Multiple Sclerosis by Cathy Chester May 17, 2017 Pgs. 1-4

[14] How to Be a Friend to a Person with MS By Madeline R. Vann, MPH and Christina Vogt
Medically Reviewed by Jason Paul Chua, MD, PhD Reviewed: October 5, 2021 Pg. 3

we love and that love us to be in our corner and in our lives. We want to pave the way for honest conversation and acceptance. We have to start somewhere; let's start with the language.

References and Resources

1. *11 Things You Should Never Say to Someone with MS. Medically reviewed by the Healthline Medical Network — Written by Ann Pietrangelo — Updated on March 16, 2016* https://www.healthline.com/health/multiple-sclerosis/things-you-should-never-say

2. *MS & Things People Should NOT Say by Ashley Ringstaff June 25, 2013* https://multiplesclerosis.net/living-with-ms/ms-things-people-should-not-say

3. *Things people say to a person with multiple sclerosis...and shouldn't by Penelope Conway from the Positive Living with MS website, November 3, 2020*

https://positivewithms.com/things-people-say-to-a-person-with-multiple-sclerosis-and-shouldnt/
4. *Supporting Someone Who has MS*
https://www.mssociety.org.uk/care-and-support/emotional-support/supporting-someone-with-ms

5. *What People SHOULD Say to Someone Living with Multiple Sclerosis by Cathy Chester May 17, 2017*
https://multiplesclerosis.net/living-with-ms/what-people-should-say-to-someone-living-with-multiple-sclerosis

6. *How to Be a Friend to a Person with MS By Madeline R. Vann, MPH and Christina Vogt Medically Reviewed by Jason Paul Chua, MD, PhD Reviewed: October 5, 2021*
https://www.everydayhealth.com/multiple-sclerosis/living-with/how-friend-person-with-ms/
7. *20 Facts About Multiple Sclerosis by Jack Kost Writer - Photographer - Advocate*
https://allegoricallittera.blogspot.com/p/blog-page_20.html

Section 6: On a Personal Note

Essay 18: Epiphanies and Truths About Me and My MS

Being faced with adversity changes you and assesses your merit. It also makes you face some truths about who you are, what you are, and who/what you want to become. Having been diagnosed with MS and having to deal with my MS has given me some insight as to who I am and what I want to become and accomplish. Here are some truths and epiphanies about myself that I have come to realize:

1. **I have not fully accepted my MS.** I was having a conversation with a friend a few days ago, and every time we started talking about my MS, I heard myself refer to MS as "my condition." Now, an "condition" is a

state of health; a "disease" is "a particular destructive process in an organ or organism, with a specific cause and characteristic symptoms." I realized that I was not in complete acceptance of my MS because MS is not a condition; it is a disease! I have an autoimmune disease, and the sooner I fully accept my circumstance, the better chance I will have to fight my disease.

2. **Non-acceptance might classify me as a hypocrite.** It also dawned on me that if I have not fully accepted my MS, then I probably have not been honest about my journey with MS. I have some reevaluating to do…. Here goes nothing….

3. **I was relieved to get my diagnosis about MS.** My health had been on a downward spiral for more than eight years; my initial diagnosis was myelopathy and positional vertigo. I did everything my first neurologist told me; from physical therapy to chiropractic to yoga – whatever was suggested, I did it. I kept getting worse, and all this neurologist could say to me was, "You have myelopathy and vertigo, I

don't know what else to tell you." This neurologist would not approve my request to see another neurologist within my current medical network, and I had to demand and fight for repeats for MRI's and spinal taps. I finally had to go to another hospital when my MRI results indicated Multiple Sclerosis, but my former neurologist insisted there was no change. It was at the other hospital that I got my true results and diagnosis.

4. **I was (and am) MAD AS HELL!** What kind of a doctor tells their patient "I don't know what to tell you," but refuses to allow you to get a 2nd opinion within their network? What kind of doctor tells you there has been no change in your condition when the results clearly state an indication of Multiple Sclerosis? What kind of doctor can watch their patient's condition deteriorate and do absolutely nothing??? I then had to ask myself the $64,000.00 question: Why did you stick with this doctor that was not helping you for so long? This question angers me more than any other

because it forces me to own my complicity in my present circumstance. Would my physical state be this bad had I trusted my gut and instincts and sought help from another sooner? The "what ifs" are driving me crazy!!!

5. **Some days I get angry and depressed.** Truth be told, it is impossible to have a debilitating disease like MS and not think about what you have lost. Me? I think about losing the ability to maintain my balance and coordination (which makes my high heel shoe collection obsolete); I think about the fact that I now walk with the assistance of a walker and not extremely far; that I can only drive short distances now and only to stores that have a pickup service because I can't walk through the stores and drive back home. Not to mention I now have bladder issues (this is not cute). Some days I feel so isolated and alone I want to scream. And, as much as I know my husband loves me and is concerned about my health and welfare, I get so upset when Carl asks me "are you okay? Are you in pain?" because pain has

become an everyday staple for me. There are days I feel like my MS sits on me like a giant weight I can't move, and I don't know which way to turn....

6. **I do not know how to ask for or accept help.** Here's the thing – I have had to be self-sustaining for quite some time. First, out of necessity as I always felt my asking for help placed a burden on those around me and then, by choice. I loved and still love my independence! But with my MS I am forced to become dependent to a certain extent, and it is awfully hard for me. I feel weakened somehow by needing help; I also know that this character flaw is to my detriment. I cannot work myself to the point of exhaustion and expect to be able to function the next day. So, I try to ask for help when I know I am going to need it as opposed to waiting until I am at the point of dropping from exhaustion. I am getting better, but I still feel like I am placing a burden on my friends and loved ones....

7. **Food is not my enemy and should not be my emotional crutch.** I am a foodie,

and I love to cook and eat. But growing up, I was taught to use food as an emotional crutch. If you had an accomplishment, you got your favorite meal. If you had an emotional upset, food was provided for comfort. I have had to undergo some real mind changes about food; again, dieting was a temporary activity, same as exercising. However, changing my eating lifestyle habits is somehow easier for me than the exercising. I love discovering new recipes and new ways to prepare the foods I eat. And, while I may backslide some days, I love healthy eating!

8. **Exercise is not the enemy!** I have said this before – I hate exercising. For me exercise was always a temporary activity to assist in my temporary weight loss episodes. Now, exercise is done to save my life. I know that if I stop moving, I will stop moving, PERIOD. So, even on days that I do not want to get up and do my walking, I make use my exercise videos (courtesy of Dom Thorpe's MS Warrior Programme[1]), I

---

[1] Dom Thorpe's MS Warrior Programme https://dt-training.co.uk/ms-warrior-programme/

extend my times with the Deb Gunter Abs Challenge[2] [3], and I do squats insofar as my knee issues will allow. It's not an easy thing to accomplish, but I am working on making exercise an integral part of my lifestyle.

9. **The right family and friends make this journey a lot easier.** The one thing about my family and friends is that they back me with everything they have! They let me know that I am loved and that they will be there to help me with whatever I need. They also are there to keep me grounded and truthful to myself, like my friend did when she so gently let me know that I was not being honest with myself about my MS. We all need people like this in our lives for checks and balances. We may not always want to hear what they have to say - we may even be resentful of their telling us — but we would not be as strong as we are

---

[2] Deb Gunter's March Commitment Abs/Core Challenge 2021 FULL ROUTINE on YouTube

[3] Deb Gunter's March Commitment Abs/Core Challenge 2021 Chair modifications on YouTube

without them, and I am truly thankful to them for putting up with me.

Truthfulness and honesty, while we do not think about them, are essential components - nay, weapons – for this journey with MS. The more we face our truths, the lighter our stress and burdens become. The old adage is absolutely spot-on: "THE TRUTH WILL SET YOU FREE!!!"

References and Resources

1. *Dom Thorpe's MS Warrior Programme* https://dt-training.co.uk/ms-warrior-programme/

2. *Deb Gunter's March Commitment Abs/Core Challenge 2021 FULL ROUTINE.* https://youtu.be/PR27R5kAuT0

3. *Deb Gunter's March Commitment Abs/Core Challenge 2021 Chair modifications* https://youtu.be/OyVB9ho-1KQ

Essay 19: Me and My MS - My Identity vs. My Fears vs. My Future Yet to Be

May 5, 2021

I'm having a rough week. I had an appointment on Monday with a pain management specialist, and Friday I will be undergoing a nerve block procedure where they will shoot cortisone into a nerve in my knee. Hopefully, this will take care of the knee pains that have been holding me back with my exercising and my walking. But in order to prepare for this procedure, there was the Monday appointment, which required walking through the Rush University Professional Building (or, at least walking to a concierge to order up a wheelchair so that I can make it through the professional building).

Tuesday, I had physical therapy (which I enjoyed because I always feel better afterwards), but Wednesday I had to have a COVID prescreening test. The only time slot they had available was for 11:00 AM. Well, my husband does not get home from work until noon, so I came up with the bright idea of saving him some time (my husband, bless his heart, has been running ragged ever since my diagnosis, becoming my chauffeur, personal assistant, personal shopper, the whole nine yards) and I decided to drive myself; it wasn't going to be that difficult. Well, it was difficult for me because my MS affects my right side and managing the gas pedal and the brake is all on the right side. It got to be a lot of stress and it was overwhelming.

I then had another epiphany: when it comes to me dealing with my MS, the reason I have such a problem is not the disease itself. It's me because I see my MS as jeopardizing my identity. I'm comparing how and who I used to be as opposed to who and how I am in this moment. When I forged my identity decades ago, I forged it based on my independence. My independence gave me self-assurance, self-reliance, a sense of power, a sense of freedom and a sense of accomplishment. I cherished that and I still cherish it. But now MS has come into my life, I question who I am and how I identify now that my independence has so dramatically diminished. If I am no longer independent, who am I? How can I be self-assured? How can I be self-reliant? How can I be ME? This fear had basically begun to cripple me - the fear of not knowing who I am now that I have MS and I can't do for myself as I used to. That is a lot to deal with.

This is terrifying for me. And I dare say, it is terrifying for anyone that has MS and begins to lose the aspect of their identity. But then I had to look at my situation again. I am still me; I'm still Carol, and I still have an identity. What I have to do is stop looking at what I am losing. The more I focus on what is negative in my life, the more inclined I am going to be to not do the work that I have to do in order to beat my MS. The final result will be that MS wins, and my fears become reality.

I'm going to be honest with you: dependence also terrifies me because, even though I am married, I do not have children. If something happens to my husband, I'll have to rely on, as the phrase goes, the kindness of strangers. The mere thought of this sends me into a panic. I am scared of what the worst could be. But then I had to realize that there is a future out there with MS that is so much brighter than I'm currently focusing on! So, let's evaluate the positives of the situation at hand. If the nerve block works, the pain will be gone, which means I will be able to walk, move, and become more independent, which also means my identity of being self-assured, self-reliant, and self-sufficient comes back.

I realized I can't dwell on the "what ifs" of life. The questions are there but they cannot be my focus – I'll "what if" myself into the crazy house! I have to focus on what I know are the possibilities of a future yet to be - a bright future yet to be. I have to work within the constraints of who I am and what I have to deal with right now. That is a given. I don't have a choice about that. This is what I have. I have MS and I have a fight on my hands. But if I do everything that I am supposed to do, everything that I know I need to do, I have such a joyous and splendid future ahead of me.

I have decided my future is going to be wonderful. It's going to be filled with the love of my family and friends. I will have my independence and I will have what God has determined I will have. Saying this, I have to give my fears to God. I cannot walk around with all of this fear in my heart and spirit. I have to give it to God and let him oversee it. I alleviate my fear by doing the work I know I must do, and I do it with an open heart and an open mind, and with the sense of creating a bright and beautiful future. I have also gone on Facebook and searched Google for support groups for MS. These groups can be a great resource of information as well as camaraderie. That is how I get through it. This is how I am going to get through.

Never let fear keep you from living your life to the fullest, getting the support you need, and doing the work you need to do.

I love you fellow MS fighters – all the way to the moon and back.